The Athlete in You

The Athlete in You
A Sportsmedicine Self-Care Guide

William F. Bennett, M.D.

Pinnacle Press ❖ Sarasota, Florida

The Athlete In You
Sportsmedicine Self-Care Guide
William F. Bennett, M.D.

Published by: Pinnacle Press
P.O. Box 2787
Sarasota, Florida 34230-2787   USA
Phone: (941) 955-8301 ~ 800-307-0001
Fax: (941) 953-3915
E-mail: pci@smallbizz.org
Internet: http://www.smallbizz.org/pci/

First Printing 1996
Second Printing 1997, revised
Printed in the United States of America

Library of Congress Cataloging-In-Publications Data
Bennett, William F. 1962-
    The Athlete In You
    A Sportsmedicine Self-Care Guide

Includes: Table of Contents, Appendix and Index
1) Sports 2) Fitness 3) Medicine 4) Health

Library of Congress Catalog Card Number: 96-069341
ISBN: 0-9647700-3-2 : $12.95

Cover design by Foster & Foster, Inc.

Dedication

With all my love, I dedicate this book to my family. My mother and father are the backbone of my success and chose, while maintaining their respective careers, to "parent" their children. One of us, may her soul rest in peace, will be unable to read this manuscript. I know, Penny, that you are with us always. Know that Tamera will have me as her guardian angel. It is my only hope that I am able to "parent" my future children equally as well as my parents.

DISCLAIMER:

This book is neither intended to replace the advice of any medical personnel nor does it guarantee the prevention of injuries. If you have sustained an injury and do not get better in a short period of time, you should seek professional medical attention immediately.

Contents

Introduction

PART 1: COMMON INJURIES BY SPORT

PART 2:   PRINCIPLES OF SELF-CARE

Foreward

Athletes are among the most challenging groups of patients to care for. Baseball pitchers repetitively throw a ball overhead at ninety miles per hour. Skiers literally fly down a mountain, and marathon runners race 26.2 miles on hard pavement in just over two hours time. These and countless other examples illustrate how athletes place tremendous stress on their musculoskeletal system. The ligaments, tendons, muscles and bones can usually support those forces if the athlete is well conditioned and is prepared for them. Unfortunately, injuries will occur even in the elite athlete if one of the components of the musculoskeletal system has failed as a result of overload.

The second challenge athletes present is that these patients demand that they return to their former level of performance as soon as possible following the injury. Athletes frequently have unrealistic expectations following their injuries and can be difficult to treat emotionally, as well as physically during the inevitable rehabilitation. These patients can also be a joy to care for, however, because they are highly motivated and will diligently work at physical therapy to overcome their injuries.

Given the athlete's obsession with his or her body and performance, I have always been surprised at how few books are available to explain in layman's terms athletes' injuries and what they can expect during the recovery phase. I could not think of any book which reviewed all of the common recreational sports, their injuries, and how the athlete could avoid them.

Dr. William Bennett has changed all of this. Bill, an orthopaedic surgeon and sports medicine specialist, has just written the "Bible" on sports medicine injuries for the layman. This book is neatly divided into three sections which allows the reader easy access to a specific question or problem. The strength of the book is the first section which uniquely describes prevention and technique modifications to avoid common injuries, *sport by sport.* The second section describes injuries and the third section outlines specific injuries and their treatment.

This book is exhaustive and is a welcome addition to sports medicine literature. **The Athlete in You** is must reading for athletes of any age and for those delivering medical care to injured athletes.

Prevention is the best treatment for all athletic injuries and is the central theme of this book.

Domenick J. Sisto, M.D.
Clinical Instructor, Orthopaedic Surgery
UCLA School of Medicine

Sports Medicine Fellowship Director
Los Angeles Orthopaedic Institute
Sherman Oaks, California

Preface

We are all athletes in our own way. Whether we participate in competitive sports, do aerobics twice a week, play weekend tennis or go bowling once a month, most of us perform some type of strenuous physical activity.

Although we may dream of stardom, most of us are not professional athletes. We do not have coaches, trainers or team doctors and sometimes are ill-prepared to get out onto the field after sitting behind a desk all week.

The result is that many athletic injuries can and do occur. Almost all injuries can be prevented. Many can be self-diagnosed and treated, while others require the attention of a doctor or specialist. **The Athlete in You** will help you navigate your way through various types of injuries, preventions and treatments of common musculoskeletal injuries.

As an active athlete, I have played a number of sports and suffered my own share of injuries. As a sports medicine doctor, I have treated many more. This book brings together my knowledge and experience as an athlete and as a doctor.

Amateurs, professionals, coaches, trainers, parents, officials, sports program administrators, physicians, physical therapists and health club personnel can all benefit from owning this quick reference guide to common athletic injuries.

Acknowledgments

I would be in no position to write this book without the years of formal training that I have been through. For the past fourteen years it seems to have been a constant uphill battle. Without the inspiration of mentors along the way, I believe the summit would have been insurmountable.

Thus, I would like to thank: Germaine Bree Ph.D.; Harry Gossling M.D.; John Fulkerson M.D.; Vert Mooney M.D.; Yens Chapman M.D.; Domenick Sisto M.D.; Roy Sanders, Bruce Browner M.D.; Christian Gerber M.D. and Philip Spiegel M.D. for their tutelage.

Introduction

The Athlete in You is divided into three sections. The first section, classified by sport, describes preventive measures and technique modification for common injuries. The second section describes the anatomy of an injury, detailing the nature of general musculoskeletal injury as well as self-diagnosis, care and "red flags," signs that indicate when a doctor should be consulted. The third section outlines specific injuries by anatomy and how to treat them.

Appendices provide a list of sports medicine societies and educational requirements for those pursuing a career in the medical field.

The methods and practices discussed in this book have helped me become a healthier person and a better athlete. I hope they can do the same for **The Athlete in You**.

PART 1:

COMMON INJURIES
BY SPORT

If you play a particular sport, you may want to learn about common injuries associated with that sport. Find your sport described in this chapter and learn how modifying your playing technique can help prevent injuries.

CHAPTER 1:

BALL SPORTS

—— ● —— ● —— ● —— ● ——

BASEBALL

Baseball is the sport with the least amount of injuries per game. However, because so many athletes play the sport, the number of injuries per year is second only to football.

Most baseball injuries and those involving the shoulder and elbow are caused by improper and repetitive overhead throwing techniques.

SHOULDER

Shoulder pain commonly results from overhead throwing. Pitchers experience this pain more than players in other positions simply because of the frequency of throws per game.

When you throw a ball overhead, you subject your shoulder to forces that can exceed your body weight. These forces develop in the different phases of throwing or pitching a ball.

During the windup, you rotate your trunk at least 90 degrees and bend your elbow at least 90 degrees as you begin to place the ball over your head.

While cocking, you further rotate your trunk and bring the ball behind your head. Your shoulder is extended and externally rotated with your elbow at least 90 degrees.

In the early acceleration phase, your arm is completely extended behind your head. Your elbow can exceed 90 degrees and your shoulder is almost completely inverted, with the back of your hand pointing towards the ground. Then during acceleration you begin to bring your arm forward and across your trunk.

In follow-through, you complete the throw and your arm continues to move across your trunk.

Most of the force across the shoulder occurs during the early acceleration phase. In fact, you can stretch out the front of your shoulder capsule. Avoidance of this injury requires that you strengthen your external rotator muscle, the infraspinatus and teres minor. Using the proper technique for throwing overhead also reduces the incidence of injury.

TYPES OF INJURIES

An improper throwing technique can cause several types of shoulder injuries. These include neurological injuries, impingement, biceps tendon injuries and shoulder instability.

NEUROLOGICAL INJURIES

Pitchers often experience compression of various nerves exiting the neck. This occurs because of their chronic muscle use, as well as the hypertrophy (the enlargement) of the muscles around the neck and shoulder. Have you ever awakened with tingling in your fourth and fifth fingers? When such tingling results from hypertrophy of muscles in your neck it is called thoracic outlet syndrome.

Try sleeping with your arm at your side. If you sleep with your arm outstretched directly overhead, you may aggravate this problem.

The fourth and fifth fingers can also become numb and tingling when you irritate a nerve around your elbow. This is cubital tunnel syndrome caused by the irritation of the ulnar nerve on the inside of your elbow. Pitchers often experience this injury.

The neck can also be a source of weakness and a cause of shoulder pain. This occurs when you have degenerative changes of discs in your neck or when the nerves that exit the neck are affected. The nerve roots that exit the neck innervate all the muscles that are used when throwing a ball. If you have shoulder pain, have a physician examine your neck.

The muscles in and around your shoulder can compress the suprascapular nerve. If you have this problem, you will likely experience pain when throwing overhead. Volleyball players also experience this injury. If you look in a mirror and notice a hollowing effect on the back side of your shoulder blade, you may have this injury.

Impingement

Experiencing pain when the arm is brought into the overhead position may be due to an impingement injury. When impingement occurs in your arm, or humeral head, the ball portion of the socket in your shoulder joint runs into the roof of the bone of the acromion. Between the ball and the roof lie your rotator cuff and bursa. These structures become compressed and inflamed.

Your rotator cuff could be called a rotator hood as it can be likened to a hood on a windbreaker. The experience of pulling the strings tightly on a windbreaker and having the hood grab your face is similar to how the rotator cuff grabs your humeral head. When the ball hits the roof, you generally feel pain from the inflammation of the rotator cuff and the bursa.

When older people have such pain, it is usually because their rotator cuff has degenerated. In younger patients, particularly pitchers, pain occurs because the shoulder is unstable.

Proper pre-game stretching, especially of the posterior shoulder, and warm-up can strengthen the rotator cuff.

Strengthening the internal and external rotators can prevent this problem. The muscles which, with your elbow at your side, rotate your hand to your belly and away.

BICEPS TENDON

Injuries can also occur to the biceps tendon inside your shoulder joint. You may recall seeing actor Arnold Schwarzenegger flexing his biceps. The tendons of the biceps muscle go into your shoulder and are inserted on the edge of the socket.

Pitchers can experience problems with the insertion of the biceps tendon because it slowly tears away from its place of insertion. This injury is known as a superior labral anterior to posterior (SLAP) lesion. Physicians can repair this injury if it is detected early.

SHOULDER INSTABILITY

When the ball portion of your shoulder travels farther forward or backward than it should, you create shoulder instability. Shoulder pain can result when your muscles cannot center the ball in the socket, which causes too much stress on the shoulder capsule.

For example, when the arm moves too much in the forward direction, the back portion of the shoulder capsule, which is circular, becomes flattened and scarred. This occurs when you thrust the ball portion of your shoulder forward and the ball hits the roof lying over the bone. The roof is curved downward in the back and the front of the shoulder.

When you experience shoulder pain, you should rest, apply ice, and use non-steroidal anti-inflammatory medications.

In general, seek the attention of an orthopaedic surgeon early. Shoulder pain caught early can usually be treated without surgery. Your physician will probably place you in a physical therapy program to stretch your posterior capsule, instruct you in proper throwing technique, and eventually strengthen the internal and external rotators of your shoulder.

PREVENTION

❖ Use an overhead throwing technique.

❖ Have someone film your pitching, then view it to see whether you are using the proper technique.

❖ Learn the proper techniques from the beginning.

❖ Thoroughly stretch your posterior capsule.

TECHNIQUE MODIFICATION

❖ Throw overhead, not sidearm. When you throw sidearm, you increase the forces across your elbow and shoulder, causing more stretching on the front of your shoulder.

❖ Make sure you follow through. If you stop early, you may cause small tears in your shoulder area.

❖ There is some controversy as to whether or not curve balls increase the stresses felt in the shoulders and elbow. They probably do not, but you should avoid this pitch if you have pain.

RED FLAGS

❖ Any shoulder pain with overhead throwing is a red flag or sign that the injury should be examined.

ELBOW

Elbow pain is common among throwing athletes, including pitchers. This pain is considered to result from improper throwing technique.

This pain occurs during the cocking and early acceleration phases of throwing. Great forces are transmitted across the elbow joint during these phases. Most elbow pain in throwing athletes occurs on the inside of the elbow.

The ligament that holds the two arm bones together can become partially torn with repetitive throwing. However, if this injury is treated, an athlete can prevent the ligament from ripping and creating an unstable elbow.

TYPES OF INJURIES

Pain on the inside of the elbow can often occur when

throwing sidearm, so athletes should avoid such throws. Injuries that occur on the inside of the elbow include medial epicondylitis and ligament tears.

MEDIAL EPICONDYLITIS

Pitchers use a number of muscles that cross their elbow on the inside of their arm. With continued throwing and sidearm pitching, they can inflame the muscles where they are inserted into the bone. If you experience pain of this type, you should rest, apply ice, and use non-steroidal anti-inflammatory aids.

MEDIAL COLLATERAL LIGAMENT TEARS

In addition to the muscles on the inside of your arm, a ligament holds the upper arm bone to the lower arm bone. With improper throwing technique, you can inflame this ligament.

With continued inflammation, the ligament can tear. All athletes, especially pitchers, need to avoid this injury. Ligament tears can result in aborting a pitching career and needing surgery.

PREVENTION AND TECHNIQUE MODIFICATION

* Throw overhead.
* Avoid sidearm throws.
* Avoid curve balls.
* Follow through.
* Use proper equipment, including pads.

RED FLAGS

* Medial elbow pain is a red flag or sign that the elbow should be examined.

OTHER BASEBALL INJURIES

In addition to shoulder and elbow injuries caused by throwing, other types of injuries can occur. These injuries can result from players sliding into a base, squatting at the catcher's mound or fielding a ball.

Injuries associated with sliding include abrasions, ankle and knee sprains, hand sprains, head injuries, and hamstring pulls. Sliding headfirst is associated with a high incidence of injury. Try to slide feet first. Proper sliding technique includes keeping the lead foot elevated, starting the slide at the correct distance from the bag, maximizing body-surface contact, and avoiding last minute hesitation.

Injuries experienced by catchers include digital ischemia, collision with runners, and meniscal injuries from crouching for long periods of time. To prevent these injuries, use a well-padded glove, avoid direct contact with runners, and stand and stretch your knee muscles often.

Injuries sustained by players fielding balls include collisions with other players and with fences, as well as hamstring pulls.

BASKETBALL

Compared to baseball players who primarily sustain injuries from repetitive motion and continued use of improper technique, basketball players' injuries result from forceful contact. Typical injuries include ankle sprains, jumper's knee, anterior cruciate ligament (ACL) disruptions, and jammed fingers. Injuries often occur in the ankle, arm, chest, elbow, foot, hand, hip, knee, leg and wrist.

FOOT

TYPES OF INJURIES

BLISTERS AND CALLUSES

The most common injuries to basketball players are blisters and calluses in the foot area. Avoid such injuries by wearing properly fitting shoes and keeping your feet dry and clean.

SPRAINS AND STRESS FRACTURES

The second most common injury to the foot is sprains to the metatarsals and stress fractures that occur from improperly padded basketball shoes. Players with high arches are predisposed to plantar fascitis which causes pain in the arch of the foot. Athletes who frequently play basketball should buy high quality shoes. Proper stretching, particularly of the gastrocnemius (calf muscle) complex, and strengthening the muscles in front of the leg can prevent sprains and fractures.

PREVENTION

* ❖ Wear well-cushioned shoes.
* ❖ Wear shoes with strong ankle support.
* ❖ Tape your ankle.
* ❖ Warm-up thoroughly.
* ❖ Stretch your quadriceps muscles.
* ❖ Strengthen the muscles around your ankle.
* ❖ Only play when rested.
* ❖ Consider using an ankle support.

ANKLE

TYPES OF INJURIES

ANKLE SPRAIN

An ankle sprain usually occurs in basketball when you land on the foot of another player and roll your foot inward. If you have taped your ankle and are wearing a strong ankle support, you will minimize the chance of turning your ankle.

If you sustain an ankle sprain, rest, apply ice, keep your hi-top shoe on, and use non-steroidal anti-inflammatory aids. Rehabilitate by strengthening and stretching your ankle.

ANTERIOR CRUCIATE LIGAMENT DISRUPTION

ACL disruption is a rare injury, but it does occur. This injury is a tear of one of the main knee ligaments and often occurs when you forcefully twist your knee. Your knee will immediately swell to the size of a grapefruit and feel unstable or give out when you walk. You may hear a pop. If you sustain this injury, you should rest, apply ice, elevate the knee, and apply a compress.

RED FLAGS

❖ Red flags are the swelling of the knee to the size of a grapefruit, instability in the knee, and a locking of the knee.

JAMMED FINGERS

A common injury among basketball players is the jammed finger. This usually occurs when you are about to catch a ball, steal a ball, or intercept a pass. The injury can also occur when someone is trying to steal a ball from you or when you turn away from an incoming ball at the last minute. Tired athletes often sustain this injury. The fingers may bend backward, causing pain and swelling.

You should rest, apply ice, and tape your jammed finger to the other fingers.

RED FLAGS

❖ Red flags include marked swelling and black and blue tissue. Severe swelling may be a fracture. You should have it x-rayed.

OTHER BASKETBALL INJURIES

Stress fractures and shin splints to the lower leg can also occur. These injuries typically result from improper shoe wear.

Older basketball players occasionally can disrupt their Achilles tendon, which is about four centimeters above their heel. Signs are a popping sound and extreme pain in the Achilles tendon and an inability to walk.

FOOTBALL

Football is another contact sport in which injuries are usually related to trauma or direct contact in spite of the use of heavy protective equipment. Some of the injuries that occur, as well as methods to prevent and treat them, are similar to those experienced in basketball. However, such injuries as ankle sprains, ACL disruptions, and jammed fingers are even more common in football.

Stinger injuries in the neck, medial collateral ligament (MCL) injuries of the knee, and turf toe are specific to the sport of football. Athletes can avoid them by wearing protective gear and modifying playing techniques.

TYPES OF INJURIES

STINGERS

A "stinger" is a sharp shooting pain, numbness or tingling down one or both arms experienced after making a tackle with your head.

When you make a tackle with the butt of your head, the normal curvature of your neck, which is curved backwards, is straightened. Then the further flexion or forward bending of the head compresses the nerves exiting the neck that innervate the neck and shoulder muscles.

PREVENTION
* Use proper padding, both helmets and shoulder pads.
* Hit with your head up.
* Hit with your face mask.
* Do not arm-tackle.

RED FLAGS
* See a physician regarding a stinger. This injury can

be serious. If such symptoms as numbness, tingling, or weakness do not quickly disappear, you should not play sports again until you have consulted your physician. Get X-rays. Multiple episodes of stingers can place you at risk to become a quadriplegic. The decision to continue the sport should be made by a professional. If you are careful, you can avoid the risk of seriously injuring your spinal cord.

MEDIAL COLLATERAL LIGAMENT (MCL) INJURIES

To prevent knee ligament injuries, select your cleats for natural grass or Astroturf. This will prevent your foot from remaining in the ground when you are tackled. In addition, use proper bracing. If you sustain such an injury, rest, apply ice, and elevate the knee.

RED FLAGS

❖ Red flags include continued pain on the inside of your knee or an unstable feeling in the knee.

TURF TOE

Turf toe occurs when you play football wearing a soft-soled shoe that allows your big toe to become caught in the turf while your body and your foot continue to move beyond your toe. This injury can be more painful than it sounds.

If this occurs, tape your big toe and wear a hard-soled shoe. Apply ice, rest, and use non-steroidal anti-inflammatory aids.

PREVENTION

❖ Wear a hard-soled shoe.

RED FLAGS

❖ A red flag is when you continue to experience pain after two weeks.

OTHER FOOTBALL INJURIES

You should wear a football helmet that fits properly. You should not be able to move or spin your helmet on your head. When your helmet fits snugly, you can reduce your susceptibility to cuts on your chin and nasal bridge.

The front guard piece should be three-fourths of an inch from the eyebrow. The back rim should not cover the occiput (the lower portion on the back of your head). Jaw pads should fit snugly on the cheek.

Even if a helmet fits properly, you can sustain a concussion. With your first mild concussion, you may return to play if you are asymptomatic after one week. After a second mild concussion, you should wait two weeks. After a third time, you should wait until the next season to play.

With your first moderate concussion, you can return to play in one week if you are asymptomatic. After a second moderate concussion, you should wait one month. After a third moderate concussion, you should not play until the next season. With your first severe concussion, you should wait one month. With a second, wait until the next season to play.

Your thumbs and fingers can become caught while tackling. Tape them to one adjacent finger to prevent this injury.

The usual ligament injuries of an ACL ligament disruption can occur. Sometimes this injury simply cannot be prevented.

SOCCER

TYPES OF INJURIES

The leg experiences high angular velocities when soccer athletes kick a ball. Thus, the leg not only experiences a great percent of all soccer injuries, but it can also be the instrument of injury.

The practice of "heading", using the head on the ball, is unique to soccer and leads to injury. When you hit the ball with the side of your head or flex your head at the ball, injuries are likely to occur. Neck fractures can also occur.

Because most soccer games involve running and kicking the ball, the foot is especially predisposed to injury. When you kick the ball with your foot pointing downward like a ballerina, much stress is transmitted across the foot in this manner. You may experience pain in the front of your ankle, known as an anterior traction injury, as well as pain in the back of your heel, known as a posterior impingement injury.

Other foot injuries include the following: ankle sprains; hallux rigidus, a condition in which the first joint in your toe becomes painful; turf toe, resulting from catching your toe in the turf; reverse turf toe, which is pain on the top of your great toe; and subungual hematomas, involving bruising of your toenails.

Such severe injuries as ligament disruptions in the knee and fractures of the lower leg bone can also occur. Refer to the chapter describing injuries by body part in Part III.

PREVENTION
❖ Wear a sturdy shoe that will not allow your forefoot to bend easily.

TECHNIQUE MODIFICATION
❖ Absorb the ball with your forehead, rather than try to hit the ball with the top of your head.

RED FLAGS
❖ Red flags are continued pain in any body part for more than a week.

VOLLEYBALL

Volleyball consists of a number of playing techniques, including blocking, passing, setting, hitting or spiking, diving, and serving. Injuries in this sport can affect almost any part of the body from the head and cervical spine to the foot.

TYPES OF INJURIES

FOOT AND ANKLE

Foot and ankle injuries are quite common among volleyball players. Ankle sprains are especially common and should be treated with ice, rest, elevation, splinting and occasionally casting. Achilles tendonitis can also occur with chronic and repetitive use. The pain usually occurs four centimeters above the heel. Stress fractures and compartment syndrome can occur. Sesamoiditis and plantar fasciitis can also occur. The primary treatments have been discussed in other chapters. Refer to the chapter on ankle injuries in Part III.

JAMMED FINGERS

Volleyball players frequently experience jammed fingers. Tape your jammed fingers.

SHOULDER INJURIES

Shoulder injuries are the most common injuries. They occur because of the continued overhead activity of the shoulder. Such injuries include impingement, rotator cuff tendonitis, shoulder instability, and suprascapular nerve entrapment.

Rather than discuss each injury, I will discuss how they occur, how they feel, and how to prevent them. All of these injuries will cause shoulder pain when you raise your hand over your head.

Your shoulder consists of a ball and a socket. However, when you move your shoulder, the ball has to move and rotate without moving upwards because there is a roof of bone over the shoulder. The rotator cuff, which is a combination of four tendons, acts to move your shoulder. At the same time, it holds the ball down and away from the roof of the bone.

If the cuff does not function properly, the ball migrates upwards and hits the roof, causing pain. This occurs when the rotator cuff is inflamed because the nerves innervating the cuff are pinched, the cuff is torn or inflamed, or the shoulder is unstable.

There are a number of different causes for the same symptom, shoulder pain. You should seek medical attention early if this injury occurs.

PREVENTION

❖ Thoroughly warm up.
❖ Stretch your shoulder thoroughly prior to playing.
❖ Strengthen your rotator cuff.

TECHNIQUE MODIFICATION

❖ Swing directly overhead, not sidearmed.

RED FLAGS

❖ The red flag is shoulder pain. An excellent stretch is to place your shoulder and elbow against a wall at eye, breast, and waist level. Then turn your opposite shoulder towards the wall. This exercise will stretch out the posterior capsule.
❖ If you are going to do such strengthening exercises, be careful to avoid strengthening your deltoid.
❖ Do internal and external strengthening exercises with your elbow at your waist. This should strengthen your rotator cuff exclusively.

CHAPTER 2:

HEALTH CLUB SPORTS

AEROBICS

Most of the injuries already discussed, except for hand injuries, can also occur in aerobics. Shin splints and stress fractures are the most common injuries. A high quality aerobics shoe can help. If you have the opportunity to choose from among several different aerobic studios, try to find one with a shock absorbing floor. Be careful with step aerobics. When you are tired, you can fall off the step and sprain your ankle.

EQUIPMENT

Nearly every day I see advertisements for exercise equipment. Soloflex, NordicTracs, StairMasters, treadmills, and stationary bicycles are just a few products being advertised.

Stationary bicycles, treadmills, and the StairMaster are exercise machines designed for aerobic exercise. With exercise of various durations and frequencies, you can strengthen your cardiovascular (heart) system.

Each type of machine involves different exercise techniques. If you purchased one of these machines for home use, follow the instructions included. If you are using a machine at a gym, seek instruction prior to starting.

This equipment is usually quite safe to use. However, with a low impact, medium-range intensity workout, repetitive motion injuries can occur.

TYPES OF INJURIES

The injuries that can occur with these devices include the following: shin splints, compartment syndromes, stress fractures, carpal tunnel syndrome, and plantar fasciitis.

Most injuries that occur during the use of the StairMaster, treadmill, or stationary bicycle affect the lower leg, feet, and hands.

Your lower leg can sustain such injuries as shin splints, compartment syndrome, and stress fractures.

Another common injury is carpal tunnel syndrome from continued compression on the surface of the palms of your hand. This occurs when you place most of your weight on your hands when grasping side-rails.

You can also sustain injuries to your feet. The most common injury is Plantar Fasciitis, an inflammation of the tissues on the sole of your foot.

SHIN SPLINTS (LOWER LEG)

Shin splints, also called medial tibial syndrome (MTS), are a common injury to the lower legs. They frequently occur when you first begin exercising on a machine. They also occur when you are a veteran of the machine who decides to increase either the interval, resistance, duration, or frequency of the exercise. The repetitive nature of exercise on the stationary bicycle, treadmill, and StairMaster predisposes you to this type of injury.

The muscles on the inner and outer parts of your leg are attached to your leg bone, or tibia, by fascia. As you exercise, this area is subjected to stress caused by muscle contractions. With repetitive contractions, the fascia can become inflamed as a healing response. Inflammation can cause pain or burning in your legs.

During exercise and with increased intensity of exercise, you may notice a burning sensation along the inner or outer shin. This burning can be severe pain that requires you to cease your exercise. An attempt to return to exercise can create the same pain. You may also experience this pain during walking.

Shin splint pain typically occurs along a line from your big toe to either the inner or outer side of your kneecap. If you experience pain at the extremes of this line, either near your ankle or near your kneecap, this is probably not due to shin splints.

PREVENTION

❖   Stretch.

❖   Warm up.

❖   Use heating pads prior to exercising.

You can use several prevention measures. Do stretching exercises prior to exercising with the stationary bicycle, treadmill, or StairMaster. Stretching loosens up muscles, tendons, and fascia in your legs. This decreases the likelihood of tearing these structures.

Stretch both the muscles in the back of your leg and in front of your leg. A stretching textbook or athletic trainer can instruct you in how to stretch these muscles.

If you have experienced this injury in the past, you may want to use a heating pack or warm soaks prior to exercise. Avoid applying ice prior to exercising. This simply tightens up the muscles and makes your leg less flexible. Wrap heating packs in towels and place them around your leg. Place the heat directly along the line from your great toe to the inner or outer part of your kneecap, depending on which side of your shin hurts.

Technique Modification

❖ Slowly increase the frequency of exercise.

❖ Slowing increase the duration of exercise.

❖ Slowly increase the interval of exercise.

❖ Exercise with your foot flat, not up on your toes.

Gradual increases in the frequency, interval and duration of your exercise will help prevent injury. However, don't overdo it. The most common cause of injury is to increase any of the above too quickly. Your body needs time to compensate for increased loads. Also try to exercise on these machines with your foot as flat as possible. Avoid exercising while standing on your toes.

Red Flags

❖ No pain relief after two weeks.

❖ Numbness or tingling.

❖ Loss of function of your leg, foot or toes.

Some other injuries mimic a shin splint. These include compartment syndromes, popliteal artery syndromes, superficial peroneal nerve entrapments, and stress fractures. Such injuries can be somewhat more disabling so you should consult a physician for an evaluation.

Compartment Syndrome (Lower Leg)

Just as shin splints can occur through repetitive exercise on stationary bicycles, treadmills, and StairMasters, compartment syndrome can also develop. However, this injury is not as common as a shin splint.

The muscles in your lower leg are not only connected to the bone by fascia, but certain groups of muscles are enclosed in sheaths of fascia called compartments. Four major compartments occur in your leg: two are behind, one is on the outside and one is in the front.

During exercise, your leg muscles undergo repetitive contractions that result in increased blood flow. This can cause the size of your muscles to increase. If you exercise regularly, you can develop hypertrophy or muscle enlargement.

When a muscle increases in size by either increased blood flow or hypertrophy, the fascial sheaths surrounding the muscles sometimes do not expand. The size of the compartment does not increase its volume, even though the muscle is trying to do so.

Within these compartments are nerves, as well as arteries that supply blood to the tissues. When your muscle increases in size, but cannot expand because of fascial restraints or compartments, the nerves, arteries, and muscles themselves can become compressed. This is known as compartment syndrome.

When the tissues in your compartments become compressed with exercise and you develop compartment syndrome, you may experience pain, numbness, or tingling in your legs.

PREVENTION

❖ Stretch thoroughly and apply heat before exercise.
❖ Stretch thoroughly after exercise and then apply ice.

TECHNIQUE MODIFICATION

❖ Slowly increase the frequency of exercise.
❖ Slowly increase the duration of exercise.
❖ Slowly increase the interval of exercise.

RED FLAGS

❖ Numbness or tingling.
❖ Loss of function of the leg, foot or toes.

If a compartment syndrome is severe, your leg and foot muscles may not function. You may have difficulty lifting your toes or ankle. You may not be able to push off when walking.

If you experience an immediate loss of muscle function, numbness, or tingling during or just after exercise, you should cease exercising and elevate the leg. Icing may help the pain, but avoid prolonged icing, as well as heating. Seek medical attention as soon as possible, preferably from an orthopaedist with sports training.

STRESS FRACTURES (LOWER LEG)

Stress fractures can occur through exercising on stationary bicycles, treadmills, and StairMasters. This type of injury is less common than the shin splint and the compartment syndrome.

Stress fractures occur from activities like aerobics and running that repeatedly require the body to leave the ground and return to the ground.

A stress fracture is a break in a bone. Repetitive cycling of the bone causes it to become fatigued and to break.

When a stress fracture occurs, you usually notice the immediate onset of pain in your leg. The pain may occur on the inside or outside, near your ankle or knee, or in your foot. The pain is often quite uncomfortable.

The pain can be quite similar to that which results from severe shin splints, so you may find it difficult to differentiate between the two injuries.

With stress fractures, you generally do not experience any numbness, tingling, or loss of function.

PREVENTION

❖ Wear properly cushioned shoes.
❖ Stretch before and after exercising.

RED FLAGS

❖ No pain relief after two weeks.

If you suspect you have a stress fracture, the self-treatment I recommend is to stop exercising, ice the injury, administer a splint, and use crutches.

If your pain does not subside in two weeks, you should consult a physician. An x-ray can determine whether or not you have this injury. Even if you have an x-ray, the fracture may not be visible on the film. Bone scans can then be used to help make an accurate diagnosis since fractures are sometimes not visible on x-rays. An orthopaedist should treat such an injury since it may require some type of immobilization, perhaps even a cast.

CARPAL TUNNEL SYNDROME (HANDS)

Carpal tunnel syndrome is another injury that can occur with the use of the treadmill and StairMaster. I have seen this injury occur more from exercising on the StairMaster than any other device.

This syndrome has many different causes. The syndrome usually occurs with activities that require repetitive use of the hands. Applying direct pressure on the palms of the hands or holding the hands with the wrist bent toward the forearm for long periods of time can lead to this injury. Typists, computer users, and laborers using jack-hammers, among others, often find themselves repetitively applying pressure to the palm of their hands either by direct pressure or by wrist position. Pregnancy can also cause this syndrome.

The palms of the hand has two large pads of tissue, one at the bottom of the little finger and one at the bottom of the thumb. Between these two pads of tissue runs the large median nerve from the forearm. The nerve extends through a tunnel, the carpal tunnel. The floor of the tunnel is bone, and the roof is a ligament, a strong band of tissue that operates like a tension wire on a bridge. This nerve lies between the bone and ligament.

Any condition that causes a decrease in the space of the tunnel or that causes direct pressure on the nerve can cause Carpal Tunnel Syndrome.

If you experience this injury, your hands fatigue quickly when you use them. The longer you use them the weaker they feel. This is usually an early sign of this syndrome. As

CTS progresses, you may notice tingling or numbness in your fingers, usually on the thumb side of your hand. You may also experience pain in your hands. With an extremely longstanding injury of this type, you may feel as if the muscles in your hand seem to be disappearing.

Following the onset of these symptoms, some people notice their hand falls asleep when they are sleeping. In fact, they may wake in the morning with their hands feeling weak or numb.

PREVENTION

❖ Do not place all the weight of your hand on exercise bars.

❖ Make sure you grasp the bars as you would railings or stairs.

❖ Avoid turning your palms upside down to support your weight.

❖ Use a weightlifting glove, one with cushioning in the hand.

TECHNIQUE MODIFICATION

❖ Place your hands facing forward.

❖ Try to avoid holding onto a railing at all.

I have developed my recommendations for technique modification on the basis of my own observations. I have treated patients who have developed Carpal Tunnel Syndrome by using the StairMaster. When I initially did not know how their injuries occurred, I suspected they were the result of weightlifting. However, many of these patients had not been engaged in weightlifting.

When I later visited a gym, I began to watch how people used the StairMaster. I noticed how they grasped the bars, which are usually angled like the railings are on stairs. They held them in a reverse direction with their fingers pointed backward and palms pointed forward. They placed much of their weight on these bars.

After observing this, I asked some of my own patients how they held their hands on the StairMaster. Many reported that they often positioned their hands in a reverse direction when their hands felt tired.

Try to avoid placing excessive weight on your hands and grasping exercise bars in reverse direction.

RED FLAGS

* ❖ The onset of weakness in your hands.
* ❖ Numbness or tingling in your hands.
* ❖ Pain at night or upon awakening.
* ❖ Muscle wasting in your hands.

If you have begun to develop carpal tunnel syndrome, avoid the activity that causes your symptoms. Sleeping with your hands in a position that does not allow the wrist to flex may also help.

If you begin to experience weakness in your hands, numbness, tingling, or pain, see an orthopaedist. Different approaches can be used to treat this syndrome. If this injury is diagnosed early, anti-inflammatory medications, rest, and splinting can help. Injections of steroids into the tunnel can sometimes help, as can surgery.

Refer to the chapter in Part III on hand and wrist injuries.

PLANTAR FASCIITIS (FEET)

Another injury that can occur with the stationary bicycle, treadmill, or StairMaster is Plantar Fasciitis. The word "plantar" refers to the bottom part of feet, "fascia" refers to the tissue inflamed in your foot, and "itis" means inflammation.

This injury also occurs through repetitive use. The injury is more common among those exercising with the StairMaster than with other machines.

The plantar fascia tissue connects the heel to the toes. The tissue acts like a boat's windlass, which is a horizontal drum on which rope is attached in order to pull up a load.

When you pull up your big toe, this action causes the plantar fascia to wind up like a windlass. With repetitive actions that cause this tissue to wind up and be pulled, inflammation can occur.

With this injury, you may experience pain and tenderness along the inside of your heel. The soles of your feet may also feel tender. With exercise, you may feel a burning sensation in the sole of your foot.

Once your plantar fascia becomes inflamed, the pain and burning are usually worse after you have been sitting for a long period of time or when you awaken in the morning. The pain or burning may subside the more you use your feet. You may also feel some numbness or tingling in areas of your foot.

PREVENTION

❖ Do a thorough warm up.

❖ Stretch your calf muscles.

❖ Strengthen the muscles in front of your legs.

The muscles surrounding your leg and ankle help to balance the ankle and foot. When you use a StairMaster, you develop the muscles in the back of your leg. Thus, you should also strengthen the muscles in the front of your leg.

You also need to strengthen the muscles in your foot. Perhaps you have seen a pulley machine with a leather harness at a gym. Place this harness around your toes and raise your ankle toward your nose. This can strengthen the muscles in front of your foot.

These techniques can help reduce the pressure on the fascia of your feet and prevent this injury.

TECHNIQUE MODIFICATION

❖ Perform exercise with your feet flat.

When you use a StairMaster, you generally stand on your toes. You do not usually exercise standing with your feet flat. Stand as close to flat-footed as possible when exercising.

Standing on your toes requires the use of the gastroc-soleus complex of muscles in the back of your legs. This complex inserts into the back of your heel. When these muscles contract, they pull up the back of your heel. The main effect is stress across the plantar fascia, the tissue between your heel and toes. With repetitive use, this tissue can become inflamed.

RED FLAGS

* ❖ No relief of pain after six weeks.
* ❖ Numbness or tingling in your foot.
* ❖ Loss of function of your foot.

If you begin to experience pain or burning along the medial part of your heel, cease exercising. When you wake up in the morning, as well as just prior to exercising, try warm soaks or heating pads. If the pain and burning remain and continue even after exercise, icing may help. The best treatment for this condition is stretching and strengthening.

If, after a period of six weeks, you are not healing, consult an orthopaedist with sports medicine training.

For more information, see the chapter on the ankle and the foot in Part III.

WEIGHTLIFTING

Weightlifting has become more popular with society's concern about having a more aesthetic appearance. I could write an entire book about weightlifting injuries and techniques to use with different weight machines and exercises. I will describe some general principles to understand.

When lifting free weights, particularly if you are new to the sport, always use a spotter-the buddy system for safety. Using free weights is different from the use of weight machines, so be careful. Free weights require that you balance the weights as opposed to relying on machines that hold weights in certain positions for you. You should also be aware that your body is using more muscles than it normally would use exercising on a machine.

Use a complete motion for whichever exercise you are performing. Avoid locking out any joint, because the load is transmitted through your muscles and then back to the joint. After that, the muscles relax, and you can injure the joint. To develop the muscles, try to stop just short of locking out. Also try to reduce your load.

Those who feel the need to lift great amounts of weight should train in this manner. If you avoid locking out, when you do perform a maximum set of weightlifts, you will be much stronger because you have isolated your muscles.

Always be conscious of your back, particularly when squatting, curling, or deadlifting. To avoid placing too much strain on your back, avoid moving your back forward during these lifts. When benchpressing, avoid arching your back. Bench-pressers are particularly predisposed to injuring their shoulders.

A small joint in your shoulder, not your true shoulder, can become inflamed when you lift. This injury can take months to heal, and even then heals only if you stop lifting. Go slowly on benchpressing, particularly on the inclined bench.

TECHNIQUE MODIFICATION

❖ Avoid lock out.

❖ Keep your back straight.

PREVENTION

❖ Always use a spotter.

❖ Consult a trainer if you do not know a particular lift.

❖ Exercise the same body part only every other day.

❖ Work your muscles, not your joints.

RED FLAGS

❖ Any unremitting pain.

CHAPTER 3:

INJURIES TO YOUR ATHLETIC CHILD

GROWTH PLATE INJURIES

The bones of children are much more elastic than those of adults. If a child sustains a great force, he is likely to injure the growth plate of the growing bone. Sprains and strains among children are less common injuries than those to his/her growth plate.

Children have two types of growth plates. All long bones have two growth plates known as the epiphysis. These are cartilaginous in nature and allow the long bones to grow. The growth plate found in the area where muscles insert into the bones is called the apophysis.

Both growth plates can sustain injuries. The growth plates in children are weaker than their bones, tendons, and ligaments. Blows children receive in various athletic endeavors can damage the epiphyses. If the damage is severe, it can disrupt a child's growth. The apophysis can also become irritated with repetitive stress. Such stress occurs because of repetitive contractions of muscles that connect directly into the apophysis. An example of this type of injury is Little Leaguers' elbow among baseball players.

Little Leaguers' elbow is most common in young pitchers. The muscles on the inside of the elbow can create excessive force across the growth plate there. To prevent it, limit the number of innings your child pitches. Stretching the inside of the elbow can also help avoid injury.

If the injury is left untreated, it can cause the end of a pitching career and lead to the growth plate's never healing. Require your child to rest if he experiences this injury.

A number of areas on a child's body can experience injuries to growth plates. When it occurs on the heel, it is called Severs disease. Because a child's bones may grow faster than his/her calf muscles, there may be abnormal force felt at the apophysis in the back of the heel. Your child may feel heel pain with activity. The best treatments are rest and stretching of the Achilles tendon and calf muscles.

You may have heard of Osgood-Schlatter disease in active children. A symptom of this is pain about three finger breadths below the kneecap. At the place where the thigh muscle tendon is attached, there is a band of cartilage that is an apophysis. The pain can be severe. The best initial treatment is rest. The child may occasionally need a cast placed across the knee to relieve the stress. A small fragment of bone can sometimes become loose and require excision.

Another source of children's knee pain is the kneecap. This pain is usually more common in females than males. The child typically has tight hamstrings, which should be stretched prior to any athletic activity. Try to control how the kneecap tracks function during exercise.

This can be done with the help of a physical therapist and through exercises directed at strengthening the inside muscles of the knee. At times, the kneecap moves too far to the outside of the knee. A soft knee brace can sometimes help control the tracking of the patella.

Gymnasts are particularly susceptible to spine injuries. These athletes place their spines in abnormal positions and under great stress.

CHAPTER 4:

MISCELLANEOUS

———•———•———•———•———

THE COMPUTER MARATHONER

Computer users are as susceptible to injury as athletes. More and more people are going on-line with the Internet.

This new found entertainment can become a marathon. How many of you have connected with America On-Line to the Romance Connection, and have spent your allowance talking to someone a thousand miles away who tells you he or she has perfect looks? If you have, you may be sending messages as quickly as you can type.

If you are truly a computer marathoner, you have experienced discomfort in either your hands or neck. In writing this book, I have had the same discomfort.

I wrote this book on a laptop computer with a keyboard that was much too small. I also sat in a terribly uncomfortable chair. As an orthopaedic surgeon, I almost prescribed a month of rehabilitation for myself. My hands felt numb and tingly, my neck became stiff, and my eyesight seemed to diminish. I learned much that I can share with you.

You may be suffering from one of many chronic overuse syndromes associated with workplace or at-home computer use.

To maintain comfort, you must avoid pain in your back, neck, hands, and elbows.

Let's begin with your chair. Solid lumbar support can help you avoid back pain. A chair that allows you to rest comfortably without bending forward or backward when viewing a screen can help you avoid neck pain.

Positioning your wrists so that you avoid bending them upward or downward to type can help you avoid carpal tunnel syndrome.

Sitting at the right height in front of the keyboard can also help. Your elbows should extend and be supported with your wrists supported at keyboard level. This can reduce extensive flexing of the elbows that can lead to compression of the ulnar nerve known as cubital tunnel syndrome.

PREVENTION

❖ Use solid lumbar support.

❖ Sit up straight.

TECHNIQUE MODIFICATION

❖ Use a wrist support so that your wrist rests in a neutral position while you type.

❖ Make sure your elbows are not too bent but are approaching the keyboard in a straight fashion.

RED FLAGS

❖ Numbness in your hand.

❖ Neck pain.

CHAPTER 5:

RACQUET SPORTS

Except for the overhand serve in tennis, the similar maneuvers of racquetball, squash, and tennis can lead to similar injuries. I will focus on the overhand serve in tennis and the smash in racquetball and squash, both of which cause shoulder pain.

TENNIS, RACQUETBALL, SQUASH

TYPES OF INJURIES

SHOULDER PAIN

Shoulder pain in racquet sports is common since athletes raise their racquets overhead. The shoulder is a ball and socket joint. Because the socket part of a shoulder is relatively shallow, the shoulder's stability depends upon its supporting and surrounding tissues.

The ball in the socket of the shoulder joint hangs below a roof of bone. When you raise your hand over your head, you must keep the ball from running into the roof bone. If, however, this occurs, you experience pain from what is known as the impingement syndrome. You then experience both tendonitis and bursitis because both the tendons and bursae are inflamed.

You can experience the impingement syndrome with the overhead serve in tennis, the smash in racquetball, and the overhead smash in squash. The syndrome is an inflammation of the soft tissue structures in the shoulder. If this injury is left untreated, it can damage your rotator cuff and cause it to tear, possibly making it impossible for perform these activities again.

Once a tear has developed, you will experience actual weakness in your shoulder. The tear can become larger if left untreated. Surgery then becomes your only treatment.

Shoulder pain should be treated early in its course. Medications and physical therapy can generally assist you in returning to play.

TECHNIQUE MODIFICATION

❖ Use proper serving techniques and properly rotate your trunk.

❖ Use preventive measures.

❖ Thoroughly warm up.

❖ Stretch thoroughly.

❖ It's especially important to stretch your posterior shoulder. Do this by bringing your arm across your body.

RED FLAGS

❖ A red flag is shoulder pain with overhead activity.

TENNIS ELBOW

The second most common injury in racquet sports is tennis elbow, as well as reverse tennis elbow. You may experience pain on the outside or the inside of your elbow when making contact with the ball.

Pain on the outside of your elbow is tennis elbow. Pain on the inside of your elbow is reverse tennis elbow, sometimes called "golfer's elbow."

Both conditions result from an inflammation of the tendons that insert into the bones around your elbow. This is a common condition and should be treated.

Rest is the best treatment, in addition to taking some anti-inflammatory medication. Physical therapy can occasionally be used to stretch the muscles in this area. You can use a splint across the elbow to immobilize the wrist, allowing the inflamed muscles to rest. Ice can also help.

Some athletes can even continue to play by tightly wrapping a strap around their forearm. The strap allows the force of the muscles to hit the strap, rather than the inflamed tendons.

TECHNIQUE MODIFICATION

* Make sure your racquet is well strung.
* Use preventive measures.
* Stretch and warm up well.
* Strengthen your elbow and wrist muscles.

RED FLAGS

* A red flag is continued elbow pain.

OTHER INJURIES

Racquet athletes also experience calluses around the hands and fingers, as well as wrist pain. Make sure your hands are always dry. When you perspire, frequently use a towel to wipe your hands. Developing a strong wrist is a way to prevent wrist pain.

CHAPTER 6:

ROAD SPORTS

BICYCLING

TYPES OF INJURIES

The most common injury to cyclists is road-rash. Bicycling clothing is usually quite thin, so it does not afford adequate protection for the skin. Cuts, bruises, and head injuries are also common among competitive cyclists.

Saddle sores are also common. With conditioning, however, a cyclist's bottom usually becomes toughened. Nerves can occasionally become compressed in the anus and the groin area. Because of the unusual seats on cycles, men especially find that the nerves around their genitals become compressed, resulting in pain and numbness in the groin and testicle area.

Cyclists can also experience numbness and tingling in their fingers when they place their weight on their hands.

Many tendons can become inflamed when riding. The Achilles' tendon can become inflamed with cyclists who sprint or stand when climbing hills.

Knee tendons can also become inflamed because of overuse. The most common knee pain comes from the kneecap. This is caused by the large number of miles traveled during training or racing. Back pain can also develop in cyclers who have a tube or center bar that is too long and forces the rider to lean and stretch too far forward. This places the back under great stress, causing it to fatigue quickly.

Competitive cyclers are predisposed to inadequate hydration and hypothermia or hyperthermia, depending on the environment in which the riding occurs.

The most effective modifications are related to the riding position and to the proper adjustment of the bicycle. The bike should be lightweight. Proper protective clothing should be worn. When standing with your legs on either side of your cycle's top bar, your groin should be one to two inches above the bar. When the bike's foot pedal is in the down position, your knee should be slightly flexed, not fully extended. A seat placed too low may predispose you to kneecap problems.

You should pedal at about ninety to 110 revolutions per minute. Slower revolutions may predispose you to kneecap problems.

PREVENTION

* ❖ Wear thick clothing.
* ❖ Adjust your cycle seat to the proper height.
* ❖ Know your weather conditions.

TECHNIQUE MODIFICATION

* ❖ Avoid placing much weight on your hands.
* ❖ Use a forearm rest.
* ❖ Use a bike with a center bar that is not too long.

RED FLAGS

* ❖ Red flags include pain and numbness in the groin or hand.

ROLLERBLADING

TYPES OF INJURIES

Rollerblading has recently become popular. Most injuries occur because of falls. Thus, the best way to prevent injuries is to wear the appropriate protective gear. This includes wrist guards, which are carbon fiber gloves that transmit force away from the wrist in a fall. Other protective devices include helmets, knee pads, and elbow pads.

RUNNING

TYPES OF INJURIES

Runners are predisposed to many irritating conditions. These include afflictions of the ankle, back, foot, hip, knee, and lower leg. Most injuries in runners are due to chronic and repetitive overuse.

Examine yourself for anatomic features that may predispose you to injuries. Increased pronation, the condition in which your ankle rotates too far inward when your heel hits the ground, can cause a number of problems, especially knee pain. This can be identified by examining running shoes you have used for some time. If the shoes are greatly worn on the inside and hardly worn on the outside, you probably have excessive pronation. Placing a wedge in your shoe can counteract the unfavorable effects of this problem.

Runners who have too much internal rotation of the hips, appearing severely knocked-kneed, or who have a wide pelvis can develop knee pain because of the great stress on the kneecap.

People who have one leg shorter than the other can especially experience pain in the hip and back.

The most common injury to the knee is to the kneecap. The kneecap can experience too much pressure from moving mobility caused by running on uneven surfaces or from poor shock-absorbing running shoes. Make sure you wear high quality running shoes. The substance used on the shoe to protect the center of your sole, called the mid-sole, is most responsible for determining the amount of pressure felt by the rest of your body.

Wear running shoes made of materials that decrease the shock to the lower leg, both compressive and shear, and that maintain resiliency (the ability of the shoe to return to normal height). Five major running shoe materials are as follows:

1) Plastazote
2) Pelite
3) PPT
4) Spenco
5) Sorbothane

Of these, Plastazote is the most effective and Sorbothane is the least effective.

These materials, on average, lose fifty percent of their shock-absorbing capacity after 25,000 cycles. They lose twenty-five percent of their capacity after fifty miles and forty percent after 250 miles. Thus, choose your shoes accordingly. Your orthopaedist may be able to assist you.

In choosing a running shoe, the most important consideration is shoe fit and comfort. Use the length-thumb rule: You should be able to place a thumb between the tip of your toe and the front of the toe box. The width-pinch rule means you should be able to grab a pinch of cloth on either side of your foot. Look for flexibility, rather than rigidity, in order to move the metatarsal break to thirty degrees.

Pain on the inside of a knee is usually caused by excessive pronation. Pain on the outside of a knee can be caused by running on uneven terrain. Pain felt deep within a knee is usually caused by stress on the kneecap.

Pain in the lower leg can indicate shin splints, fractures, and the compartment syndrome that occurs when the lower leg muscles expand and compress the nerves. Doing sufficient stretching and avoiding overuse, as well as using well-padded running shoes, can prevent these injuries.

The foot can also sustain a variety of strains. For more information on injuries to the lower leg and foot, refer to the chapters on these body parts in Part III.

PREVENTION

❖ Use a high quality running shoe.

❖ Change your shoes regularly.

❖ Examine an old pair of shoes for abnormal wear.

TECHNIQUE MODIFICATION

❖ Run on a different road or path each day.

❖ Run one time clockwise and the second time counterclockwise.

❖ Stretch well.

RED FLAGS

❖ Red flags include pain in the feet, knees, and lower legs.

CHAPTER 7:

STICK SPORTS

— ● — ● — ● — ● —

CRICKET

Cricket, a combination of lacrosse and baseball, is a common sport in the United Kingdom. Propelling the ball is called bowling, and catching the ball is called fielding.

TYPES OF INJURIES
While injuries in cricket can occur anywhere, they generally occur in the back and shoulder. Back injuries occur because of the abnormal forward-leaning position used when trying to stop the ball. The shoulder is also subject to pain because of impingement, which was described in the earlier chapter on tennis and other racquet sports.

PREVENTION
❖ Muscle flexibility.
❖ Muscle strengthening.
❖ Cardiovascular endurance.

TECHNIQUE MODIFICATION
❖ Always use the proper techniques.

RED FLAGS
* ❖ Any cricket injury can be a red flag.

GOLF

The wrist, back, and shoulder are the limbs most frequently injured in the sport of golf. The best way to prevent these injuries is a combination of proper conditioning and understanding swing mechanics. Taking golf lessons can be helpful.

TYPES OF INJURIES

HAND AND WRIST INJURIES

The hand and wrist can experience strain to the tendons and ligaments. A bone in the lower inside of your hand can cause pain when your hand engages in repetitive swings or experiences abnormal impact with the ground. In general, a period of rest, anti-inflammatory medication, and icing can reduce your symptoms.

Golfers can experience pain on both the inside and the outside of the elbow. Such injuries are usually caused by inflammation of the tendons around the elbow.

Treatment for these injuries is divided into four stages. First, address the inflammatory process by resting, applying ice, administering anti-inflammatory medications, and splinting. Second, strengthen the forearm muscles to increase their flexibility and endurance. Third, decrease the force felt by the wrist. Try using a larger golf grip. A tennis elbow strap may also help by dissipating force into the strap instead of the elbow. Curved grips may also help, and graphite clubs transmit lower force through the shaft. Finally, injecting the wrist with a steroid solution may be helpful.

Back Injuries

Probably the most common golf injury occurs to the lower back. Great force is transmitted through the back when swinging a golf club.

An effective stretching routine is important, as is strengthening the abdominals and the back muscles. The best way to prevent injury is to take golf lessons to learn proper swing mechanics. In addition, use a general conditioning program that includes developing muscle flexibility, strength, and endurance.

Prevention

❖ Stretching.

❖ Strengthening.

❖ Endurance.

Technique Modification

❖ Use a larger grip.

❖ Use a graphite club.

❖ Use a curved grip.

❖ Use proper swing mechanics.

Red Flags

❖ A red flag is continued pain after true rest.

ICE HOCKEY

Types of Injuries

Most injuries in ice hockey occur during games even though players spend approximately four times longer in practice. Most injuries are by direct contact. The most commonly injured body parts are the knee, shoulder, and groin.

Most hockey injuries occur during high-speed collisions.

This includes collisions among players, as well as collisions between players and the puck, the sticks, the ice, and the rink. Most injuries to the upper body extremity are caused by direct contact.

The lower extremity of the body is subject to many injuries, including fractures, sprains, and strains. Knee guards are only mildly effective in preventing shin injuries.

Ankle sprains are infrequent because hockey skates provide stability to the ankle. One unique injury is a laceration to the ankle tendons when sharp blades from another skater hits the exposed front part of the ankle. Protect yourself with an ankle guard.

PREVENTION
* ❖ Condition your body.
* ❖ Use proper protective equipment.

TECHNIQUE MODIFICATION
* ❖ Try to keep your hockey stick below your shoulders.
* ❖ Respect your opponents.

RED FLAGS
* ❖ Any injury can be a red flag.

LACROSSE

TYPES OF INJURIES

Lacrosse is also a game in which most of the injuries occur because of direct contact or collision. The lower extremity is commonly more affected than the upper body. In general, there is body-to-body contact, stick-to-body contact, and body to playing surface contact.

PREVENTION
* ❖ Use proper protective equipment.

TECHNIQUE MODIFICATION
* ❖ Respect your opponents.

RED FLAGS
* ❖ Any injury can be a red flag.

CHAPTER 8:

STUDIO SPORTS

—————•——————•———————•————•———————

BOXING

Professional and amateur boxing are popular in the United States and abroad. Professional boxing is far more injurious than amateur boxing.

In professional boxing, blows to the head are worth more points than blows to other body parts. The object is to render the opponent neurologically incapable of continuing to fight.

In amateur boxing, all blows are equally weighted. The bouts are shorter, and boxers are required to wear head-gear. Officials in amateur boxing are also likely to terminate a fight sooner than in professional boxing. In addition, if a fighter is knocked out or a fight is stopped because of a technical knockout, the boxer is suspended from fighting for a specified period of time.

All boxers should undergo a pre-fight examination that includes the head, eyes, ears, nose and throat, and heart, as well as a neurological exam.

TYPES OF INJURIES
The most common injuries among boxers are to the hand and wrist. Proper gloves and wrist strengthening, as

well as proper punch mechanics, can prevent fractures and sprains to the wrist and hand.

Neck injuries, while feared, are actually quite rare.

Among the common head injuries are those to the eye. The compressive forces caused by a punch to the eye are great. The intense force can affect eye pressure and cause retinal detachment.

Measures to prevent ocular injury include having an annual ophthalmologic exam, participating in a national ocular injury database development program, using a thumbless glove, educating ringside physicians about the nature of ocular injuries, and observing mandatory minimal ocular requirements.

One of the most serious injuries is to the brain from the great force and repetitive nature of boxing punches to the head. Such punches can cause cerebral bleeding and concussions. Some people use the term "punch-drunk" to describe a person suffering the effects of repetitive punching. If you have ever heard a long-time boxer speak, you have observed the effects of boxing injuries.

The medical term for punch drunk is Chronic Traumatic Boxer's Encephalopathy or CBTE. Symptoms include one or more of the following: a chronic amnesic state from scarring, which can produce short term memory loss; dementia, a progressive disorganization of personality traits; morbid jealousy, in the form of accusations of infidelity against a boxer's wife; rage reaction in which boxers display extreme violence; and psychosis involving delirium and paranoia.

PREVENTION

❖ Have educated ringside physicians.
❖ Require mandatory suspensions for knockouts.
❖ Use serial screening to look for CBTE.
❖ Have acute life support available.
❖ Decrease the length of competitive matches.

TECHNIQUE MODIFICATION

❖ Avoid boxing without wearing proper gloves.

RED FLAGS
❖ Red flags include delirium, forgetfulness, and violence.

DANCING

As you might guess, dancers most frequently injure the lower body extremity. Ballet dancers have a high frequency of injury. This is because of the extreme positioning of the lower extremity needed to perform routine ballet maneuvers.

Dancing classic ballet involves five positions. The first position requires dancers to place their heels together with their knees pointed outward and their feet in line. The second position differs only in that dancers' knees are not together. The third position requires dancers to place one foot in front of the other. The fourth position involves placing one extremity in front of the other in a position similar to that of the third position. The fifth position involves placing the feet facing each other.

Other positions include the demi-plie, the grand plie, and demi-pointe and full pointe positions. Arabesque and grand jete are two other positions requiring dexterity.

These extreme positions subject the lower extremity to injury, especially if there is an inadequate stretching program.

Poor pre-season conditioning, inadequate warm up, and lengthy high intensity training predispose dancers to injury. To condition the body for ballet, dancers should strengthen the muscles in front of both the leg and ankle, as well as those in the back of the leg and ankle.

TYPES OF INJURIES

The most common error in dance is not rotating the hip completely to ninety degrees of external rotation. Dancers often compensate by increasing the arch in their back, which predisposes them to back injury. They also compensate for the lack of external rotation by screwing the knees, which places undue pressure on the knees. They often use excessive pronation, or rolling the foot inward, to simulate the external rotation lacking in the hip. This causes undue pressure on the mid-foot.

Some anatomic features of the body type of dancers can prevent them from reaching the proper positioning. For example, dancers who do not have complete external rotation of the hip will automatically be predisposed to injury for the reasons previously discussed. If dancers have too little external rotation of the lower leg bone in relation to their knees, they may never succeed in placing their knees over their feet for the classical basic positions. Some back-kneeing is fine. However, too much of it places undue pressure on the back of the knee, which can cause leg and knee pain.

The toes of dancers assuming the demi-point position must achieve ninety degrees of motion. If not, the great toe can experience pain. In addition, because of the need for extreme positions of the ankle, dancers can experience pain in the fronts and backs of the ankles.

The back of a dancer is also predisposed to injury because of the extreme arching of the back to compensate for the inadequate external rotation of the hips.

PREVENTION

❖ Stretch well.
❖ Strengthen the muscles in the front and back of your leg and ankle.
❖ Use the proper floor for shock absorption.

TECHNIQUE MODIFICATION

❖ Use proper positioning of the lower extremity without compensatory movements.
❖ Work to achieve full external rotation of the hips.

❖ A red flag can be any unremitting pain in the lower extremity or back.

GYMNASTICS

Most of the studies of injuries among gymnasts are focused upon female gymnasts. Injuries occur most frequently during floor exercises, followed by activities on the uneven bars.

TYPES OF INJURIES

The most common injury is ankle sprain. Another common injury is tearing of the skin. Wrist injuries also occur because of the hyperextension of the wrist joint that occurs during many routine activities. Shoulder injuries, including the impingement syndrome, also occur. The feeling of pain resulting from the arm being held overhead is similar to the pain experienced in the impingement syndrome. Back injuries occur because of the great amount of force transmitted throughout the back.

PREVENTION
❖ Tape your ankles.
❖ Use a wrist block to keep your wrist from extending.
❖ Warm up well.

TECHNIQUE MODIFICATION
❖ Use proper techniques.
❖ Use a spotter.

RED FLAGS
❖ Red flags are pain in the knee, wrist, and back.

WRESTLING

Wrestling is among the sports with the highest injury rate. Injuries occur by direct blows, friction, twisting, and indirect forces.

TYPES OF INJURIES

The knee is the body part most frequently injured. Refer to the chapter on the knee in Part III to learn about the injuries that occur to the lower extremity of the body. Wrestlers can sustain any of these injuries.

Two other common injuries are cauliflower ear and impetigo. The ear is subjected to repetitive blows because of the close proximity of each wrestler's body. The ear can become inflamed and enlarged, losing its normal contours.

Wrestlers continuously experience skin scratches and cuts that can easily become infected.

The more significant health problems of wrestlers are related to weight loss. Many wrestlers who want to lose weight try to eliminate water and reduce body fat by not eating. The extreme methods some wrestlers use to lose weight predisposes them to health problems.

In general, you should wrestle at five to seven percent body fat to avoid health problems. You should completely avoid the use of diuretics, laxatives, and self-induced vomiting. Weight loss should not exceed one to two pounds per week. A balanced diet is imperative. Your weight should be managed so that you can eat a meal the night before a match. Replenish the body with fluids immediately after competition weigh-in.

PREVENTION

❖   Use high quality head-gear.
❖   Use clean wrestling mats.
❖   Lose weight gradually.

TECHNIQUE MODIFICATION

❖ Learn to fall and roll.

RED FLAGS

❖ Red flags include skin rashes, swollen ears, dizziness, and lightheadedness.

CHAPTER 9:

WATER SPORTS

—●——●——●——●—

JET SKIING

Jet skiing has become a popular sport, particularly in warm climates.

TYPES OF INJURIES

The injuries that occur depend on the type of machine used. Jet skies, wave-runners and others each have different riding positions. Machines that you sit on, require that you place your legs on either side of a seat that is usually slanted outward. This causes your knees to bend and rotate in an abnormal way. Rotational stresses can cause pain on the outside of your knee.

You may need to modify the ski seat. Narrow the seat to take away the slant that causes your legs to spread outward.

Reckless driving can cause a collision resulting in almost any injury. Always wear a lifevest. An unconscious person cannot swim.

PREVENTION

❖ Use a narrow ski seat.
❖ Use a lifevest.

❖ Narrow your ski seat.

SURFING

A sound understanding of wave mechanics can help surfers avoid injuries. Waves are, for the most part, caused by winds that create ocean swells. A wave breaks when it encounters ground resistance.

For example, the large waves formed on the north shore of Hawaii result from swells traveling for thousands of miles in deep water. The first obstacles they meet are the reefs immediately off shore. Thus, these waves have much more force than the waves around the continental United States. Waves around the U.S. are usually broken up somewhat off shore because of the continental shelf.

Wave forms are indigenous to the coast upon which they break. Surfers should study how waves break along the coast on which they are surfing.

TYPES OF INJURIES

Most surfing injuries are caused by surfers making body contact with their boards or with a coral reef. The side of a surfboard causes the most injuries.

Surfers are susceptible to contusions, lacerations, and sprains.

PREVENTION
❖ Study the surf, the ocean's bottom, tides, and the traffic.

TECHNIQUE MODIFICATIONS
❖ Take surfing lessons.
❖ Surf with a companion.
❖ Avoid the path of oncoming surfers.
❖ If you fall behind the board, try to fall on your feet or buttocks.

❖   Attend to lacerations because of the abnormal bacterial flora from the sea that can invade wounds.

SWIMMING

TYPES OF INJURIES

The most common injury experienced by swimmers is the shoulder injury known as swimmer's tendonitis. This inflammation of the rotator cuff occurs among competitive swimmers who overwork their shoulders by swimming great distances. When the shoulder becomes fatigued, the ball in the shoulder joint rides up and abuts the acromion. The major function of the rotator cuff, in addition to rotating the shoulder, is to keep the ball from moving beyond the overlying acromion.

Fatigue is not the only cause of the inflammation of the rotator cuff, commonly called impingement. An inflexible shoulder is another cause. The most important motion during swimming is the extreme position attained when the shoulder is held as if pitching a ball. If you are unable to place your arm in this position, you are probably predisposed to injury.

Another cause of the inflammation, though it might seem strange, is a shoulder that is too lax. If someone says you are double-jointed, your shoulder may be too lax. The ball of your shoulder may ride up to impinge upon the acromion.

Other injuries include pain to the front of the foot that occurs with the kick during the backstroke. An exercise program to stretch the tendons in front of the foot should prevent this injury.

The knees can suffer from strains to the inside of the knee or from medial collateral ligament (MCL) strains. Knee injuries occur primarily with the breaststroke.

Be particularly careful to avoid back injury when arching the back for the butterfly.

PREVENTION

❖ Gradually decrease your distance.

❖ Gradually increase the severity of your workout.

❖ Warm up properly.

❖ Engage in vigorous initial workouts.

❖ Strengthen muscles.

❖ Stretch well.

❖ Study proper stroke mechanics.

TECHNIQUE MODIFICATION

❖ Try to avoid excessive internal rotations of your shoulder after you reach overhead.

❖ Avoid overwork.

RED FLAGS

❖ A red flag is unremitting shoulder pain.

WATER SKIING

TYPES OF INJURIES

Water-skiing injuries, including a variety of sprains and strains, as well as contusions, can occur from falls. Skiers who fall can collide with their own skis or with boats. They occasionally become entangled in ski ropes. Injuries involving boat propellers occur infrequently.

Practicing safety around water and boats is the key to preventing many of these injuries. Always wear a lifevest even if you are an expert skier. The driver of your ski boat should be knowledgeable about nautical rules and skilled in driving boats.

Skiers use specific hand signals to communicate with boat drivers. Both drivers and skiers should be aware of such signals.

An injury specific to waterskiing is the vaginal or rectal douche. This occurs with falls when you squat on the skis. I can say from my own experience that this injury is uncomfortable.

Ear pain should also be a concern. Skiers occasionally fall head first, and the force of the water can cause a disruption of their eardrum. The back is especially prone to injury among those who do ski jumps.

PREVENTION

❖ Ski with knowledgeable boat drivers.
❖ Know hand signals.
❖ Observe water and boating safety.

TECHNIQUE MODIFICATION

❖ Take water-skiing lessons.
❖ Stand straight while skiing.

RED FLAGS

❖ Any injury can be a red flag.

WINDSURFING

TYPES OF INJURIES

The most common injury among competitive windsurfers is back injury. This easily occurs when the wind catches the board, and you try to counter the force by pulling backward with your back.

The practice of leaning too far forward to lift a sail from the water can also injure your back.

PREVENTION

❖ Strengthen the back muscles.
❖ Develop back muscle flexibility.

TECHNIQUE MODIFICATION

❖ Pull the sail with your back straight.

CHAPTER 10:

WINTER SPORTS

—————•————•————•————•————

SNOW BOARDING

Snow boarding is quickly becoming one of the most popular winter sports. Injuries among snow boarders are similar to those experienced by other skiers. The only exception is thumb injuries since there are no poles used in snow boarding. The best way to avoid injuries is to learn how to fall.

SNOW SKIING

TYPES OF INJURIES

There are different types of skiing, including ski jumping, cross-country skiing, telemarking, and downhill skiing.

SKI JUMPING

Ski jumping is probably the most dangerous form of skiing. The knoll or jump is usually about twelve feet higher than the slope. Skiers hit the ramp at speeds of about sixty-five miles per hour. When a ski jumper takes off, he must thrust his body over the front of the skis and land in a crouch, usually with one foot in front of the other.

As you might expect, the most common injuries to jumpers are bruises, fractures, and ligament tears. Preventing some of these injuries requires jumping in good weather conditions and having a well-groomed slope for take-off. Resorts have recently modified the transition zones for landings so that they are not as flat, allowing for an easier landing.

CROSS-COUNTRY

Cross-country skiing is a physically demanding sport The technique consists of a diagonal stride, a kick, and the placement of a pole, followed by the placement of the second pole. The sport requires great endurance and muscular strength. The most commonly used muscles are those in the groin and around the hip. Thus, these muscles are susceptible to strains and pulls.

The ski bindings worn by cross-country skiers must permit unrestricted motion of the knee, allowing a skier almost to walk on their skis. The front of the foot is held bound to the ski; the rear of the foot is free. Thus, in twisting falls, the foot may not release, predisposing you to injuries of the knee and ankle.

Sprains and strains are typical in cross-country skiing. Abrasions and contusions are found more often in downhill skiing.

PREVENTION

❖ Keep your feet a shoulder width apart.

❖ Stay on the trail.

❖ Be in good condition.

TECHNIQUE MODIFICATION

❖ Use proper skiing techniques.

TELEMARKING

Telemarking is a type of skiing that looks like cross-country skiing on a downhill course. In fact, the technique is similar to cross country in that the heel is free.

A telemarker must turn using great quadriceps muscle strength and rely on the poles to initiate turns. When such skiers use their poles extensively and make many turns, they place their thumbs at risk for injury, particularly if they place their wrist through straps. If their ski poles are caught in the snow, the wrist can move forward past the pole and the thumb can be caught on the pole. When the thumb is stressed, its ligaments can become sprained or torn.

TECHNIQUE MODIFICATION

❖ Avoid placing your hands through wrist straps.
❖ Wear special gloves to avoid this injury.

DOWNHILL

Downhill skiing requires specific gear, boots, skis, and poles, as well as the proper warm clothing. Thumb injuries can occur in downhill skiing in the same way as they do with telemarking.

One dangerous injury inherent to downhill skiing is catching the inside edge of your ski. The caught ski continues forward while you squat and your leg moves out and away from your body on the inner edge, while the other leg remains under your body. The attached leg travels out in front of you and at a higher speed than the rest of your body. This movement predisposes you to an injury of the anterior cruciate ligament (ACL) inside your knee.

If you sustain this injury, you may actually hear a pop. Your knee may also swell to the size of a grapefruit. Sometimes, however, the pain actually subsides and you are left with a swollen, unstable knee. Avoid skiing again. If the ligament is torn, the knee has little or no stability.

PREVENTION

❖ Take skiing lessons.

❖ Know your terrain.

❖ Know your weather.

❖ Engage in conditioning.

❖ Avoid placing your hands through the wrist straps.

RED FLAGS

❖ A red flag is a swollen, unstable knee.

PART 2:

PRINCIPLES OF SELF-CARE

This section contains self-care techniques, definitions on basic anatomy, and information on when to consult a physician (and what type).

CHAPTER 11:

INITIAL SELF-CARE

Having just finished my daily stretching and warm-up routine and straining under the heavy iron bar in my grasp while benchpressing at a local gym, I heard, "Hey, Doc, can you look at my shoulder?" I smiled to myself since this was not the first time such a request had been made. I cut my repetitions short to oblige my gym companion.

I was barraged with questions regarding his recent injury. "Well, Doc, I hurt it last night, and you know I did exactly as you would have told me. I placed some warm towels on it." (I thought to myself, "Now, this is not what I would have told you.") However, I allowed him to continue. "Did I do what was right? Do I need a splint? Can I lift again? When should I ice it? When can I play tennis again?"

Just after this recent encounter, I realized that athletes like my gym companion need to know how to administer some self-care for their newly-acquired injuries. I felt sure many athletes with injuries simply do not know if they should apply ice or heat.

Whenever I was working out, I also noticed that certain techniques used by athletes had the potential to cause injury during their work-out. I again thought about what I could do to help them.

I decided that athletes need information about how to avoid needless athletic injuries. This is why I decided to write an easy-to-follow book about self-care for athletic injuries.

THE NATURE OF INJURIES

You may wonder why pain occurs, why your limbs swell, and why an injury hurts more when you move your limbs. Pain and swelling are usual responses to any injury.

When you first injure your body, whether it be a sprain, a fracture, or tendonitis, your body tries to heal the injured tissue. The healing process normally begins with inflammation. The body tries to recruit certain substances to the injured area to help break down the injured tissue and initiate a healing response.

Some of the substances attract pain mediators (substance "P") that stimulate the nerves in the body to send messages to the brain. You decipher this message as pain.

Remember that pain is a self-defense mechanism. If a movement causes pain, you should not do it. If you continue using a body part that becomes injured, you can further injure it.

When tissues are injured, they release fluids. This is what causes swelling. The more severe an injury, the more swelling and pain occur.

SELF-CARE METHODS

In the early phases of an injury, the most common symptom will be pain, and the most common sign will be swelling. Thus, your initial self-care efforts should be directed at controlling pain and swelling.

In general, when you injure yourself, apply the principles of rest, ice, compression, and elevation (R.I.C.E.), regardless of the type of injury.

REST

If you injure yourself and continue with activity, you can injure the tissue to a greater degree than you initially did. Consider even mild pain as significant.

ICE

Many athletes believe warmth will be the best treatment for an injury because it feels good. Within the first twenty-four to forty-eight hours following an injury, the best treatment is ice, not heat. By applying ice to your body extremity, you will accomplish several goals.

First, you will decrease the amount of swelling. Icing decreases the amount of fluid that leaves the membranes of the injured tissues. Swelling can increase the pain you experience. By decreasing the amount of swelling, you decrease the amount of pain.

Second, icing, if applied properly, can create an analgesic affect. Apply ice cautiously since you can freeze your tissues and receive frostbite. When you apply ice, avoid placing the ice directly on the skin. Place the ice in a plastic bag and wrap the bag in a towel. Then place the towel on the injured limb until you feel your extremity is beginning to feel numb.

All you need is twenty to thirty minutes of ice at a time. Once your limb feels numb, remove the ice. Once the analgesic affect wears off, reapply the ice.

Use this technique intermittently for the first twenty-four to forty-eight hours. After the first twelve hours, you can decrease the frequency with which you apply ice. Your pain should decrease with the analgesic effect of the ice.

Again, apply ice instead of heat since heat causes an increase in the swelling and accentuates the inflammatory process. While the heat may feel good, you may actually experience more pain.

COMPRESSION

By compressing the injured tissue, you can also decrease the swelling, and therefore, the pain. You do not need to push on the injured tissue to achieve compression. You should also compress the injured tissue evenly. This can best be done with an ACE bandage wrapped evenly and firmly around the injured body part. You want to avoid making the compressive dressing so tight as to cut off your blood supply. If you are unsure of how to do this, have a professional do it for you. If you wrap your injured tissue and your pain increases, you should loosen the dressing.

ELEVATION

By elevating your injured body part, you can also decrease the swelling, thus decreasing the pain. Elevate the extremity above the level of your heart. Elevation allows the fluid released from your tissues to drain to your heart instead of accumulating at the injury site.

Some of my patients often think that it is sufficient to place an injured ankle up on a footstool. However, this does not elevate the ankle above the heart.

The R.I.C.E. formula applies to virtually all injuries you may sustain. You should apply it immediately when you are injured. R.I.C.E. is an early intervention strategy that can be beneficial in the long term.

If you have injured a body part in your lower extremity, rest may include using crutches until your injury heals or until you see a health professional. If you injure your arm, rest may include the use of a sling. By decreasing the weight on your injured limb, you allow it to rest.

Rest can sometimes include the use of a splint or brace. If you have any of these devices at home, apply them to your injured extremity. This will help immobilize the injured part, thus helping to rest it.

Having thus embarked on an early road to recovery by applying these basic principles of self-care, you may want to learn about symptoms and signs of injuries to pinpoint your injuries.

THE DIFFERENCE BETWEEN SIGNS AND SYMPTOMS

The symptoms of an injury can be considered your complaints. This does not mean you are a whiner. A symptom refers to the way you describe your injury. For example, consider the following scenario. You played basketball and landed on your opponent's foot. Your foot rolled over, and you experienced pain. You then heard a pop and your ankle swelled to the size of a grapefruit. Now when you walk on uneven ground your foot feels like it is going to roll over because it's unstable.

Symptoms are a description of an injury. The symptoms you experienced were pain, a pop, a swollen ankle, and the feeling your ankle might roll over. Symptoms not only can help you determine what your injury may be, but can also help your physician formulate an opinion.

Signs of an injury are what you find when you look at and touch your injured body part. If you were to visit a medical professional, you would have a physical examination.

A physical exam generally includes observation, palpation, range of motion testing, strength testing, nerve and artery testing, and specific diagnostic testing. The actual results of the exam are called the signs of an injury.

SIGNS

OBSERVATION

You can observe your injured body part for swelling, discoloration (black and blue), and any gross abnormalities that may be present. These signs indicate an injury. The more swelling and discoloration you have, the greater the severity of the injury.

PALPATION

You can palpate (touch) your injury to identify areas that are tender. This can help you determine where to apply ice. You may find more than one tender area. This is typical, since many structures can be injured.

RANGE OF MOTION

You can determine if your injured body part has a range of motion similar to the opposite non-injured part. If there is a smaller range of motion than the opposite side, this, too, indicates a significant injury.

STRENGTH

You can compare the strength of your injured body part to that of your opposite non-injured part. If the strength on your injured side is less than on your non-injured side, this may also indicate an injury. Sometimes pain reduces normal strength.

NERVE AND ARTERY TESTING

You may not be able to determine if specific nerves and arteries function. However, you do know whether you have numbness or tingling in your body part. These signs indicate that one of the nerves in the area of the injury has been affected. You can also make an indirect assessment of the blood supply to the injured area by looking for normal capillary refill. If you press on the skin nearest the injured body part, the skin should turn white or blanche. Within three to five seconds, your skin should turn back to its normal pink hue.

If it takes longer than five seconds for the pink hue to return, there may have been some damage to one of the arteries surrounding the injury. However, if the injured body part is cold, the capillary refill may be delayed.

SPECIFIC DIAGNOSTIC TESTS

Diagnostic tests should be conducted by a health professional for an accurate assessment. Some simple tests for various injuries are described in Part III, Common Injuries by Body Part.

Let me illustrate the signs of an injury. If you have twisted your ankle, you may notice that every time you walk, your ankle becomes swollen. Pushing upon certain areas of your injured ankle may cause you pain. If you replicate the injury mechanism, by rolling your foot inward, your ankle may feel unstable or feel like it is going to go out of the socket. The visible swelling, the tenderness, and the movement of your ankle in response to pressure are all signs.

SYMPTOMS

The most common symptoms that occur with injuries are as follows.

PAIN

Pain associated with injuries can range from mild to severe. The more severe the injury, the more pain you have. People differ, however, in their pain tolerance, so this is a relative judgment. You will usually experience pain at the time of the injury and may continue to experience it with subtle movements.

NUMBNESS

Numbness associated with an injury usually implies you have injured a nerve or a structure close to a nerve. Simply stretching a nerve can give you numbness. You can occasionally tear a nerve. If you dislocate a joint and a nerve lies nearby, you can also stretch the nerve.

Loss of Function of a Body Part

When you injure a body part, you may not be able to move it. The part you have injured has torn or is not in its proper place, or you are simply experiencing too much pain.

Tingling In A Body Part

Tingling in a body part suggests you have injured a nerve. This symptom is similar to numbness. However, numbness usually indicates a more severe injury has occurred.

Night Pain

Pain that causes you to awaken in the middle of the night may be related to an injury you have sustained. If you have not had an injury but experience pain that wakes you, you might have an illness not easily detectable and should see a physician.

Unexplained Fevers

Unexplained fevers with pain in a body part also suggest you may have an illness, so see a physician.

Unexplained Severe Weight Loss

If you are not actively trying to lose weight but have lost a significant amount of weight, see a physician.

Joint Dysfunction

Your joint may give out on you.

Locking

You may experience body parts locking into position.

Popping

You may hear a popping sound.

Most Common Signs

Numbness

You may have numbness in a body part.

DISCOLORATION
Your injured body part is discolored, turning black and blue.

SWELLING
You have a body part that swells to the size of a plum or grapefruit.

LOSS OF FUNCTION
You have a loss of function of a body part.

ABNORMAL APPEARANCE
A body part may no longer appear normal but it may be pointed in the wrong direction.

MUSCLE WASTING
When you have muscle wasting, your muscles seem to be disappearing.

LACK OF BODY PART MOVEMENT
You have a body part that remains in only one position.

BODY PART DISLOCATIONS
You have an ankle, elbow, knee, or shoulder that you are sure dislocated and popped back into position.

UNUSUAL MOVEMENT
You push on a body part and it moves more than you would expect.

TENDERNESS
You push on a body part and it feels tender.

Now that you have this information, and perhaps have administered some self-care, you can read further about specific injuries in Part III.

CHAPTER 12:

THE ANATOMY OF AN INJURY

Injuries usually occur when you subject your body to abnormal movements or when you perform a usual motion with excessive force or speed. With most injuries, the tissues in your body have either been stretched, torn, or broken. Before we discuss what structures you can injure, you should be familiar with some terms.

DEFINITIONS

ARTHRITIS
When you injure the cartilage of a joint, you may develop arthritis. Arthritis is a term used to refer to joint irritation that has existed for a long period of time.

Inflammation of cartilage can, over time, cause a breakdown of more cartilage and underlying bone. This can cause pain. The root "arth" refers to the joint and "itis" means inflammation.

ARTICULATION
Articulation occurs when two bones contact one another

and their cartilage ends, ligaments, and anatomic bony configuration allow them to glide smoothly.

AVULSION

Avulsion refers to an injury that occurs because of a stretching force. An avulsion injury can occur when a ligament or muscle detaches from a piece of bone.

BREAK

Bones break when the continuity of the bone is disrupted. A break can occur at the epiphysis (end of the bones), the metaphysis (part between the end and the shaft), or the diaphysis (shaft of a long bone). A small break is a fracture.

BURSITIS

When you overload a bursa, the sac between tendons and bones, you may injure its lining. Increased loads or many repetitions can cause cell membranes to release substances that create inflammation. This can cause pain.

CHONDROMALACIA

You may experience chondromalacia when you injure the cartilage of a joint. The root "chondro" refers to cartilage, and "malacia" means sick. This, too, is a type of inflammation. This condition occurs before the inflammation and breakdown of your joint cartilage has reached the underlying bone.

Chondromalacia may, in reality, be early arthritis. However, it does not always lead to arthritis.

DISLOCATION

A dislocation is a severe dislodging. For example, instead of the ends of the long bones moving slightly, they may lose complete contact with each other. This occurs because you have probably torn the capsule and some or all of the ligaments surrounding your dislocated joint. Cartilage damage can occur.

EDEMA

When any tissue is torn, there is a release of fluid into the tissues. The result is edema or swelling.

EFFUSION

When a joint becomes injured, the cells in the joint make too much fluid or effusion.

FASCIITIS

Fasciitis is inflammation of the fascial tissues.

FRACTURE

See "break."

HEMARTHROSIS

Hemarthrosis occurs when blood in the joint results from an injury to the lining of the joint or from a tear in the capsule or a ligament of a joint. The root "hem" refers to blood, "arth" refers to joint, and "osis" refers to the problem.

INFLAMMATION

Inflammation is the body's response to an injury. When you disrupt a tissue during an injury, the cells break their cell membranes. The body then releases substances to try to aid in the healing process. The substances try to attract other cells to bring nutrients to the injured tissues. The substances released to attract such cells also cause the nerves to be stimulated and tell your brain you have pain.

MYOPATHY

Myopathy refers to any muscle disease.

MYOSITIS

Myositis is an inflammation of the muscles.

NEURITIS

Neuritis is an inflammation of a nerve.

NEUROPATHY

Neuropathy means a disease of the nerves.

PULLED MUSCLE

A pulled muscle is actually a number of small tears. This injury generally causes pain and can become inflamed. Pulled muscles usually heal with time. The medical term for a pulled muscle is a strain.

SIGN

A sign is a physical finding that indicates an injury.

SPRAIN

A sprain means a stretching or tearing of ligaments. There are three different types of sprains, from mild to severe. A mild sprain is a term for a stretched ligament, whereas a severe sprain means there has been a complete tear. In between mild and severe sprains are partial tears of a ligament. Both partial tears and complete tears can cause your joints to move abnormally.

STRAIN

A strain is a pulled muscle resulting from many small tears of your muscle. This can cause pain and some muscular weakness.

SUBLUXATION

Subluxation is a condition in which your joints move abnormally. When the surfaces of the ends of your long bones are subjected to abnormal forces, they may move away from each other. When this occurs, you may stretch or tear the capsule and ligaments or injure the cartilage of the joint.

SYMPTOM

A symptom is a complaint about an injury or evidence of

an injury.

Synovitis

Synovitis is an injury to the lining of your joint that results in inflammation. The root "synov" refers to synovium and "itis" refers to inflammation. This can cause pain, as well as lead to the process of the deterioration of joint cartilage.

Tendonitis

Tendonitis is an inflammation of the tendon. When you injure a tendon, the body responds with inflammation. "Tendon" refers to the injured tissue, and "itis" means inflammation. This condition can cause pain.

<u>PAIN</u>

Pain is a normal consequence of an injury. Consider pain a natural warning mechanism. Many injuries occur when we ignore initial mild pain and keep moving, only to suffer a more severe injury with greater pain.

With most injuries, the tissues in your body will release a substance (i.e. bradykinins or substance "P"). This stimulates the sensory nerves in your body to send a message to your brain cortex. You decipher the message as pain.

There are different tissues in your body that can be injured: muscles, ligaments, tendons, bones, nerves, and joints.

Muscles

You do not have to be Arnold Schwarzenegger to have muscles. Even the skinniest person has many muscles.

Muscles are contractile tissues that move your body when they are activated. Muscles consist of many fibers made up of many fibrils. Contained in the fibrils is protein, the actual engine of the muscle.

MUSCLE BIOMECHANICS

A muscle contracts to cause movement. Generally, it shortens through what is called concentric contraction. An example of a concentric contraction is a biceps curl.

In addition, through isometric contraction, a muscle can contract without shortening. Pushing against a wall is an example of an isometric contraction.

Finally, through eccentric contraction a muscle can exert a force while actually becoming longer. An eccentric contraction occurs when a muscle contracts to slow down a moving body part. For example, when you are running and your leg is swinging forward, your hamstring muscles in the back of your leg contract eccentrically. They control your legs forward motion.

MUSCLE BIOCHEMISTRY

Proteins are the engine of your muscle. The proteins actinin, myosin, and tropomyosin, in conjunction with calcium, are the components of muscle fibril that cause muscular contractions.

Muscle contractions begin when the brain sends a nervous signal to a muscle. When the signal reaches the muscle, the body releases calcium that stimulates the three proteins to move, causing a contraction.

Between the actinin and myosin proteins are bridges that look like the arms of a spider. They contract and cause the bridges to move.

MUSCLE FIBRIL

Injury to any muscle can cause pain. After an injury, any muscle movement can be uncomfortable. This pain can range from mild to severe and can be quite disabling. You may also feel like your muscle is weak. Injuries to muscles are generally strains, small tears in the muscle. Muscle strains occur more often with eccentric contractions than with concentric or isometric contractions.

Ligaments

Perhaps you have heard someone say, "Boy, you are double-jointed!" They are referring to the ligaments or fibrous tissues that connect bones to each other. Ligaments are usually found around the joints in your ankle, elbow, hand, wrist, hip, knee, and shoulder.

Ligaments insert into your bones, where they are firmly attached. If you had no ligaments, the bones of your joints would not be held in any configuration. By holding joints in a specific fashion and providing them stability, ligaments allow bones to move around each other.

Fibroblasts are the living cells within ligaments. They secrete collagen that allows ligaments to stretch without breaking. With undue stress or abnormal motion, ligaments can stretch or tear, either partially or completely.

The severity of a ligament's injury determines how much a joint will be affected. You may experience joint instability or pain. Your joints may begin to make a clicking sound because the normal gliding motion of the joint is disrupted.

Depending on the joint and ligament that are injured, as well as the extent of the injury, you may need no medical attention or you may need your ligament repaired or reconstructed. With many ligament injuries that remain untreated, the abnormal motion creates the possibility of joints becoming arthritic.

Tendons

The terms ligaments and tendons are often used interchangeably. However, these two structures have different functions. Ligaments and tendons attach muscles to bones, and attach bones to bones.

Tendons are found at the ends of each muscle where they are inserted directly into bones by fibers called Sharpey's Fibers. Tendons allow contracting muscle tissue to pull a bone through a relatively resilient cable. Tendons, while part of the muscle complex, are not contractile tissue. That is, they do not contract.

The cells of a tendon are called fibroblasts. They secrete a substance called collagen that allows them to stretch without breaking. Tendons can, however, stretch and tear as a result of excessive force or overuse.

BURSAE

My grandmother complains about her bursitis. What she is complaining about is an inflammation of the bursa, or the protective tissue whose fluid lubricates bones. The bursa's fluid allows tendons to glide in close proximity to the bone without fraying. This is necessary because when tendons usually approach bones at an angle they may rub on them.

However, when the bursa works overtime, it becomes inflamed. This is called bursitis, which is painful.

When a tendon stretches beyond its normal excursion, you may experience a strain or a complete tear. A strain is a small tear that can create pain. If the tendon tears completely, you may be unable to move the body part you have injured because the cable has become disrupted.

BONES

The human body has two-hundred and six bones. Bones in your extremities usually connect with another bone at a joint, for example the knee joint.

Cartilage covers the end of a bone that connects with another bone. Cartilage allows each bone to glide smoothly against the other, providing shock absorption. The area between the ends of the bones and the shaft is flared.

Osteocytes are living cells in bones. These cells secrete calcium hydroxyapatite and collagen, the non-living portion of the bone. Calcium hydroxyapatite is what makes bones hard. Phosphorus also contributes to the composition of a bone.

At some time, you may have examined a skeleton. This bone is non-living because it has no living cells. The bone appears hard and rock-like. However, the bones in your skeleton, while hard, are also flexible enough to bend when force is applied to them. This is why your bones do not break when you experience the effects of gravity on a daily basis.

If a great amount of force is applied to your bone, however, it may break. The direction with which force is applied to a bone will determine whether or not it will break. Fractures are breaks of bones that can be either partial or complete breaks. Stress fractures are bone breaks that occur because of chronic loading of the bones.

If you sustain an injury to a bone, it may be a fracture, a stress fracture, or a contusion, a bone bruise. You will experience pain that is usually sudden with onset.

JOINTS

Joints are the place of union between one bone and another. They are held together by ligaments and the capsule. The major joints that I will discuss include those in the ankle, back, elbow, hip, knee, neck, shoulder, and wrist.

Ligaments like the medial collateral ligament (MCL) can be found on the outside of your joint. Those like the anterior cruciate ligament (ACL) can be found inside your joint.

The knee joint has a unique tissue called the menisci: the medial and the lateral. Menisci are half-moon shaped cartilage. They increase the surface area of a joint and provide shock absorption. The only other joint in your body with a meniscus is your acromioclavicular joint, one of your four shoulder connections.

A joint is stabilized by its capsule, ligaments, muscles, and negative pressure. The atmospheric pressure inside your joint is negative because it is lower than that on the outside. When you crack your knuckles, you allow the pressure inside your joint to be equalized to the pressure outside your joint. Cracking your joints is not usually harmful for you, but I recommend you avoid doing so routinely.

Joints held together by ligaments are covered and surrounded by a capsule. On the inner surface of the capsule is your synovium. Synovial tissue has cells that secrete the fluid found inside your joints. The fluid lubricates the joint and provides nourishment to the cartilage.

The joints of your body are covered with cartilage. Chondrocyte cells in the cartilage secrete collagen, glycosaminoglycans, hyaluronic acid, and proteoglycans. These substances combine to provide a smooth surface upon which your bones can glide. Such substances are similar in function to oil for your car engine.

Cartilage also provides shock absorption. Nourishment to most substances of your body comes by way of blood vessels. Cartilage does not have blood vessels, so it receives its nourishment from the joint fluid.

There are two ways to injure cartilage. If you sustain an injury to your ligaments, you can move your joints in an abnormal way that indirectly rubs away your cartilage. You may also directly injure your cartilage from compression.

When you injure cartilage, you sometimes experience pain. The medical reason for this pain is not well understood. What is known, is that with such an injury substances that are given off as they are with injuries to muscles and other soft tissue injuries, interact with nerves in your body. They then send an impulse to your brain that you decipher as pain. However, cartilage has no nerve endings.

Cartilage must provide for shock absorption in an orderly manner. When cartilage is injured, the bone behind the cartilage senses the abnormal forces. A sensation of pain occurs because bone has nerve endings. A cycle of continued cartilage deterioration may result if it is not halted.

Physicians may recommend you take aspirin or Ibuprofen, an anti-inflammatory medication, to disrupt this cycle. Such medications counteract the pain throughout stages of the enzymatic cycle.

If joint injuries are severe, pieces of cartilage can occasionally break off and float around inside your joint.

Your synovial tissues, the lining of your joint, can also become inflamed. This condition is called synovitis. When the synovium becomes stretched, the body releases substances that cause inflammation.

Inflammation is a normal part of the healing process. While it may cause pain, it also brings in nutrients to repair injured tissues. Injuries can occur to any of the tissues outlined above.

DIAGNOSING INJURIES

When you injure yourself, you need to make a diagnosis. You will know what body parts you have injured, but the injury you identify may be one of several diagnoses you could make. This book is designed to help you make a diagnosis.

If you choose to consult your physician regarding an injury, he or she will try to make a diagnosis by following a routine process.

First, the physician will record a history of how you injured yourself, where you feel pain, what activities increase or decrease the pain, and the nature of your complaints or symptoms. Second, the physician will perform a physical examination to check for tenderness, abnormal motion, appearance, strength, and tenderness, to assess your neurovascular status. If the diagnosis is still in question, the physician may order laboratory and other clinical tests. These may include blood work and x-rays, as well as possible bone scans, computerized axial tomography (CAT) scans, and magnetic resonance imaging (MRI) tests.

Physicians use x-rays (radiographs), to see bones. X-rays do not show cartilage, joints, ligaments, muscles, or nerves. However, physicians can infer facts about these structures from x-rays.

Bone scans are tests that require a radioactive substance to be injected into your blood. This substance identifies areas of injury. Physicians can then see such areas more clearly with an x-ray image. The radioactive level of these substances is generally not harmful. Some patients are allergic to the dye that can harm their kidneys, but there is only a slight incidence of this.

A CAT scan is an x-ray technique that allows physicians to view cross-sections of bones. Traditional x-rays present longitudinal images of bones.

MRI tests depict tissues, as well as bones. For example, physicians using MRI tests can see cartilage, joint configurations, ligaments, and muscles.

Once all testing has been completed, your physician should be able to identify your injury and recommend treatment. Surgery is not often required with musculoskeletal injuries. Bracing, using physical therapy, resting, strengthening, stretching, and taping can often be used for treatment.

SURGERY

Your injury may occasionally require an operation. With the rapidly expanding field of orthopedic surgery, minimally invasive operative techniques have been developed. Arthroscopy and laser surgery are two examples.

Arthroscopy is a technique that allows your joints to be visualized by the physician placing a small telescope into your joint. This is done through a portal or small incision about an inch in length through which the arthroscope is placed. With one or two additional portals, the surgeon can place instruments into your joint to repair injured structures.

The use of laser surgery in orthopedics is available but limited. Lasers help surgeons work on difficult-to-reach structures in your joints.

CHAPTER 13:

THE MECHANISM OF AN INJURY

—————•——————•——————•——————•———

You can generally injure yourself in three ways: acute trauma, chronic overuse, and fatigue. Several additional factors can also predispose you to injury.

ACUTE TRAUMA

Acute trauma injuries occur suddenly and without warning. Acute injuries can include dislocations, fractures, sprains, strains, and subluxations (dislocations). They can damage bones, joint cartilage, ligaments, muscles, or tendons.

Once, while trying to qualify for the Olympic wrestling trials, I tried to use a hip throw. At the same time, my opponent tried to throw me. To break my fall, I placed my hand out to my side. As I hit the mat, I dislocated my elbow. This is an example of an acute injury.

Other causes of injury, whether they be torques (twisting injury) or direct blows, can occur. No single mechanism alone causes a specific injury to a specific body tissue. The amount of force and direction of force on a body part determine what structure becomes injured.

CHRONIC INJURIES

Chronic injuries occur when you have been participating in an athletic endeavor for a period of time. Chronic injuries are not caused by a single force affecting a body area but by the cumulative effect of forces.

You generally have some indication that you may be developing an injury. For example, you may experience mild pain in a certain area of your body but continue to participate in sports.

With chronic injuries, every time you move a part of your body in a certain direction or subject it to a specific force you may experience small tissue tears. Such tears may be so small that the resultant pain is not disabling.

However, if you continue participating in your sport and sustain more tears without allowing time to heal, you can cause even more serious injury to the tissues. The longer you allow the process to continue, the higher your risk of sustaining more serious injuries. If the inflammation process continues indefinitely, you may sustain a complete tear of the injured tissues.

You can deal with injury from chronic overuse at any time, whether it is from mild pain and strain or severe pain and tearing. For example, when you play tennis frequently and for long periods of time, you may be hitting a number of backhand shots. With each shot, you subject your elbow to forces that on a one-time basis are not sufficient to cause injury. However, when you frequently play long games of tennis, these individual forces add up, perhaps predisposing you to develop tennis elbow (a tendonitis on the outside of your elbow).

FATIGUE

Both acute and chronic injuries occur more often when you first begin to exercise or when you are tired. At the beginning of an exercise session, you may try to exert yourself without having had a sufficient warm-up period. Because your body experiences the effects of sudden forces without a warm-up, your ligaments, muscles, and tendons may not be prepared to handle such forces. Injury can occur.

When you are fatigued from participating in activity for a long period of time or from a lack of sleep, you are prone to injury. When you are tired and try to exercise, your brain may tell your body to respond in a certain way, but your body may not respond or may only respond slowly.

Fatigue can cause injury in this way. Proprioceptors, or nerve endings in your joints, normally send messages to your brain about how the joints are positioned in space. For example, when playing basketball, you do not have to tell your foot to be positioned to return to the floor after a rebound. The proprioceptors send this message without your awareness of the message.

However, when you are tired, this mechanism does not function properly. Messages are sent slowly or not at all. Thus, you may fail to make a simple move like positioning your foot in the proper way. Your brain tells you, instead, to position your feet in an abnormal way, predisposing you to turn your ankle.

For your information, law enforcement officers check for proprioceptive ability when they instruct potential alcohol abusers to perform psychomotor tests. Alcohol can affect your proprioceptive abilities. Thus, if you exercise under the influence of alcohol or drugs, you may predispose yourself to injury.

ADDITIONAL INJURY

PREDISPOSITION FACTORS

EQUIPMENT

You should always use the proper sport-specific equipment. This can include such protective devices as eye protection, helmets, and protective padding, as well as such sport-specific shoes as cleats, golf shoes, or running shoes.

With contact sports like football and hockey, it is probably self-evident that protective devices like helmets and pads should be used to prevent injury.

Runners subject themselves to repetitive loads on their lower extremities. They should always wear cushioned running shoes that can absorb the force placed on the lower extremity. The surfaces on which they can run include dirt, grass, sand, and tar. Such surfaces can be flat, non-uniform, like cross-country track courses, or slanted.

If you were to run on tar with dress shoes, you would realize that this could injure you. Always make sure you have cushioned running shoes that can absorb the force you place on your lower extremity.

If you are unsure about the proper equipment needed for your sport, consult a sporting goods store manager or any experienced player. In fact, with certain activities, there may be rules that only allow you to participate with the proper equipment.

ENVIRONMENT

The environment in which you play your sport can also be a factor in avoiding injuries. When you play football on Astroturf, the cleats you wear should be different from those you wear on natural grass.

In addition, adverse environmental conditions can increase the likelihood of injury. If you play outdoor basketball games, you should be cautious regarding the slick nature of the playing surface.

Play football on Astroturf or natural grass. Play indoor basketball on a clean, dry floor. Prior to skiing, you should be aware of such important environmental conditions as clouds, fog, and ice.

You should, in addition, have people available to act as spotters or coaches, particularly with activities like gymnastics or tumbling.

STRETCHING

With any athletic endeavor, you should perform a thorough stretching routine prior to any activity. If you are like me, when you arrive at a court, on a field, or on the slopes, you are ready to play. You may also be with friends who are eager to play.

Resist the temptation to begin playing. Warm up for at least fifteen minutes. Include this fifteen minutes in the time you have planned to play. Warming up is extremely important.

Avoid bouncing when you stretch. Bouncing may cause you to experience small tears in the muscle you are trying to stretch. If you simply stretch your body continuously, the tissues in your body will expand slowly without tearing.

Stretch all parts of the body, regardless of what type of sport you play or what body parts you plan to use. I have often seen basketball players stretching their legs. They should also stretch their entire body, including their arms and shoulders. I have seen some of them sustain injuries to their arms when the opposing player tried to steal the ball or when their arms became entangled with those of another player during a rebound.

If you do not know how to stretch, consult any athletic trainer or obtain a book on stretching. Organize a total body stretching routine. Practice this routine daily until it becomes second nature. Always perform it just prior to athletic activity. Once you have developed a routine, you can then add stretching exercises to develop the specific body parts you use during your sport.

If you have access to a sauna, steam room, or whirlpool, you can begin loosening up in these facilities. You can even begin stretching there. However, if you use these facilities to warm up, remember that the environment in which you play your sport may be cooler. There is a risk of your body's cooling down prior to engaging in activity. Thus, continue to maintain your flexibility until you begin your sport.

A low intensity warm up can include an aerobic activity. For example, you may want to use the Stairmaster, stationary bicycle, or treadmill for fifteen minutes. Thus, your total warm up, including stretching, would be thirty minutes. With your blood already flowing, you have slowly increased the load on your heart and lungs. This may also be beneficial to you before you participate in your sport.

STRENGTHENING

You should begin a general strengthening routine if you plan to participate in sports for any period of time. Such a routine will develop the strength of your entire body.

After developing a general strengthening routine, you can develop a sport-specific routine. For example, if you are a bowler, you may want to develop the muscles in your forearm, hand, wrist, and upper arm. By developing strength in these areas, you can help prevent tendonitis in these areas.

TRAINING TECHNIQUES

Sport-specific training techniques should also be used. Refer to Part I, Common Injuries By Sport, for more information about individual sports.

For example, baseball pitchers should be trained to avoid using a sidearm pitch. This technique can subject the elbow to abnormal forces, predisposing one to injury. To prevent this injury, pitchers should throw overhand.

Practice is also part of training. Practice if you plan to play your sport regularly. Your practicing should be done at a time different from your game. Devote time to practicing techniques that you may later use during your game.

For instance, volleyball players should train themselves during practice sessions to develop proper techniques for bumps, serves, spikes, blocks, and sets. If they only play the game, they may never fully develop such techniques, predisposing themselves to injury.

CHAPTER 14:

SERIOUS INJURIES AND TYPES OF PHYSICIANS TO CONSULT

There are times you may seriously injure yourself. In this case, you should neither try to treat yourself nor delay seeking professional medical advice. You should know the symptoms and signs to help you determine when you have sustained a serious injury.

SIGNS

What you actually discover about your body is as follows:

- ❖ You have severe swelling of a body part.
- ❖ You have a body part that becomes severely discolored, generally black and blue.
- ❖ You have a loss of function of a body part.
- ❖ Your ankle, elbow, knee, or shoulder goes out.
- ❖ You have a body part that remains in a fixed position.
- ❖ You have an ankle, elbow, knee, or shoulder that you are sure was dislocated and then popped back into position.

In general, if any injury does not seem to be healing over a period of seven to fourteen days, see a physician.

SYMPTOMS

Your complaints are as follows:

❖ You feel an unexplained numbness or tingling in a body part.

❖ You experience pain so severe you cannot move.

❖ You suffer a loss of function of a body part when you try to move it.

❖ You notice one of your joints has given out.

❖ You sense one of your body parts locks into position and you cannot move it.

❖ Your shoulder feels like it is dead when you move it.

❖ You heard something pop when you injured your body.

TYPES OF PHYSICIANS
TO CONSULT

You may wonder what type of doctor to consult. Many types of medical professionals are addressed as doctors. The degrees and certificates earned by these professionals vary, depending on the content and duration of their academic and training programs.

Allopathic and osteopathic doctors are the only two professionals considered to be complete physicians. To qualify as a complete physician, one must have finished four years of professional training involving the study of medical care for all bodily systems. After medical school, one also completes an accredited residency ranging from three to seven years and has received the certification (Diplomate) for his/her board.

The following is a description of some of the various kinds of doctors.

ALLOPATHIC

Allopathic doctors earn the Medical Doctors (M.D.) degree and are what most people think of when they think of physicians. The term allopathic is not usually used by these doctors. The term is used more by osteopathic doctors who wish to differentiate between the two.

CHIROPRACTORS

Chiropractors are doctors who treat disorders through manipulation and spinal realignment and who earn the Doctor of Chiropractics (D.C.) degree. They cannot prescribe medication or perform surgery.

DENTISTS

Dentists treat diseases of the teeth and can have one of two degrees, a Doctor of Dental Science (DDS) or a Doctor of Dental Medicine (DMD).

DOCTORS OF PHILOSOPHY

These doctors are professionals who have received the highest academic degree for scholarly activity. They have earned the Ph.D. for studying the philosophy of their subject matter.

OPTOMETRISTS

Optometrists can prescribe glasses and contact lenses and earn the O.D. degree. They are different from an ophthalmologist who has an M.D. degree.

OSTEOPATHS

Both allopathic and osteopathic doctors are physicians. Their training is similar except for the type of medical school they attended. In addition, osteopaths perform some manipulation. Osteopaths earn the Doctor of Osteopaths (D.O.) degree.

PODIATRISTS

Podiatrists are physicians who treat diseases of the feet and who earn the Doctor of Podiatric Medicine (D.P.M.) degree.

For more information about these professionals, consult the Appendix A.

This book is devoted to athletic injuries to the musculoskeletal system. For such injuries, you will likely want to consult a physician who has either an M.D. or a D.O. degree. In addition, it is helpful if the doctor you consult specializes in sports medicine.

Sports medicine is the application of the knowledge and skills of a medical practitioner to the treatment of injuries experienced by physically active people, particularly those engaged regularly in organized sports.

Because there are no rules regarding the use of the term sports medicine, some physicians who have not completed any specialized training in sports medicine may classify themselves as sports medicine professionals.

A variety of physicians may indicate they are sports medicine specialists. These may include emergency medicine doctors, family practitioners, general practitioners, internists, orthopaedic surgeons, pediatricians, and rheumatologists.

There are professionals in non-physician groups who can be involved in sports medicine. See Appendix A.

Some physicians also may have completed additional training in sports medicine. However, if you are not consulting an orthopaedist, you are missing the opportunity to visit with a physician whose entire training has been devoted to the musculoskeletal system.

If you decide to consult a physician for a medical opinion regarding a sports-related injury, you should consult with the physician who has the most training in the musculoskeletal system. This is usually an orthopaedist who has completed additional training (a fellowship) in sports medicine.

If you decide to consult a physician for a medical opinion regarding a sports-related injury, you should consult with the physician who has the most training in sports medicine. Some orthopaedists who specialize by body part may also have an interest in sports medicine. For Example, the orthopaedic sports medicine fellowship.

Orthopaedic fellowship in sports medicine are a relatively new way of acquiring expertise in athletic injuries. Thus, there are some orthopaedists associated with the American Orthopaedic Society of Sports Medicine (AOSSM) who have no formal training in sports medicine because they were the originators of this subspecialty. (See Appendix A for information about AOSSM). Orthopaedists practicing sports medicine who have not completed a formal fellowship, may practice the subspecialty of orthopaedic sports medicine by demonstrating expertise in the field.

There are professionals in non-physican groups who can be involved in sports medicine. See the Appendix A.

Thus, though there are many who call themselves sports medicine doctors, you should initially consult with a professional with the most training in the musculoskeletal system, and one who has completed added training in sports medicine. By doing so, you can be assured of an accurate diagnosis of your injury and prompt treatment. An orthopaedist who feels you would be best served by an alternative caregiver will provide you with a referral.

PART 3:

COMMON ATHLETIC INJURIES BY BODY PART

———— • ———— • ———— • ———— • ————

This section addresses such common injuries as fractures, sprains, strains, and various types of inflammation.

To use this section, you must first determine what body part you have injured. Then turn to the relevant chapter. Injuries to a particular body part are identified by the type of injury: fractures, inflammation, sprains, and strains.

Each subsection describes the structures that have been injured, provides suggestions about what to do and what to avoid regarding self-care, and lists some of the red flags for each injury.

CHAPTER 15:

THE ANKLE AND FOOT

This chapter deals with injuries common to the ankle and the foot.

When you examine your foot, you notice that between your leg and your foot are two bony bumps. One bump is on the inside, and one is on the outside. Injuries surrounding this area, including the back part of your heel, are injuries to the ankle. Any injury that occurs lower than the ankle area is a foot injury.

Injuries to your ankle and foot can be classified as fractures, inflammation, and sprains. Fractures and sprains are usually acute injuries that occur suddenly through one incident. Tissue inflammation is usually chronic, occurring over a period of time. Inflammation occurs as a result of the increased frequency or intensity of exercise.

If you have injured your ankle or foot in one incident, most likely you have sustained a fracture or sprain. If you have been participating in an athletic endeavor and notice a gradual onset of pain and a loss of motion over time, you are feeling the effects of inflammation, generally due to repetitive overuse.

Determine if your injury is acute or chronic, and refer to the appropriate subsection of this chapter. See the sections on fractures or sprains for acute injuries, or the section on inflammation for chronic injuries. Within each subsection, you will learn about the structures you have injured, what you should do or avoid doing, and when you should see a physician.

You sometimes actually break one of the bones in your foot or ankle when you roll your ankle over. If this is the case, read the descriptions of fractures and sprains for both the ankle and the foot to determine the most likely injury. The advice regarding what to do and what to avoid is similar for both injuries.

For example, if you are playing basketball, football, racquetball, volleyball, or any sport in which you roll your ankle over, most likely you have sustained a sprain. If you experience pain and swelling around the ankle, turn to the section on ankles. If the pain and swelling are lower than the ankle, you should refer to the subsection on the foot.

If you have been running for long distances, or playing multiple sets of tennis or games of basketball, and feel pain in your ankle (including the back of your heels), turn to the appropriate section under inflammation. If the pain is lower than the ankle, turn to the description of inflammation in the subsection on the foot.

THE ANKLE

ANKLE FRACTURES

The same inward rolling of the foot on the lower leg bone that can cause an ankle sprain can also cause an ankle fracture. However, greater force is usually needed to fracture a bone. The determining factor is the rate of the applied load or force.

When a fracture occurs, you immediately experience severe pain and swelling and may hear a crack as opposed to a pop. The pain is usually quite severe, so you will be unable to walk.

At times, it is difficult to differentiate between a fracture and a sprain, particularly a severe ankle sprain and a mild fracture. With both injuries, you will have pain and may be unable to walk. An x-ray is usually required to identify the injury.

As with an ankle sprain, you should apply the R.I.C.E. formula with ankle fractures. Crutches may also be needed. You should have an x-ray of your ankle. If you have a splint, apply it to your ankle. If you suspect you have a fracture, see an orthopaedic surgeon.

OSTEOCHONDRAL FRACTURES

When you sprain or break your ankle, you may also sustain an injury to the cartilage that overlies the bones of your lower leg and your foot. The cartilage covers the ankle joint. Alone or in combination with a piece of underlying bone, the cartilage can chip off, creating a loose body in your ankle joint.

You will need an MRI to make a diagnosis of this injury. This lesion will generally cause you continued pain even after your primary injury has healed.

DO

❖ Rest, apply ice, use compression, and elevate the limb (R.I.C.E.).

❖ Use crutches, if necessary.

❖ Elevate your injured limb above the level of your heart.

❖ Use any over-the-counter non-steroidal anti-inflammatory medication, only if you can tolerate aspirin. In general, this medication should not be used until forty-eight hours after an injury.

DO NOT

❖ Continue your sport.

❖ Put heat on your injured limb.

❖ Use an anti-inflammatory medication immediately.

❖   Strangulate your injured limb with compression.

❖   Elevate the limb by placing your foot on a stool.

RED FLAGS

❖   Severe swelling

❖   Severe dislocation

❖   Abnormal movement of bones

❖   Inability to walk within a few days

ANKLE INFLAMMATION

Two main areas around your ankle can become inflamed with exercise. Achilles tendonitis can occur four finger breadths above your heel bone. Retrocalcaneal bursitis can occur directly over your heel bone.

ACHILLES TENDONITIS

Achilles tendonitis is an inflammation of the tendon of your achilles. This area is named after Achilles, a character from Greek mythology. He was indestructible, except for his heel. When it was injured, he was defeated.

The Achilles tendon attaches the gastrocnemius and soleus calf muscles to your heel bone. When your calf contracts, the tendon causes your foot to press downward against the floor.

This tendon can become inflamed as a result of exercises that require repetitive motions, high frequency, short intervals, and long durations. Because the Achilles tendon does not have a good blood supply, with repetitive use, your tendon can become inflamed. When this happens, you will feel pain in the back of your heel. The pain, generally limited to an area three finger breadths above the heel, may require you to cease your activity.

If you experience this problem again, apply the R.I.C.E. principles. In addition, wearing higher heeled shoes during the interim will help reduce the pain. Such shoes reduce the load on the calf muscle and Achilles Tendon. If your injury does not heal in a few weeks, consult your doctor.

DO

❖ Rest, apply ice, use compression, and elevate the limb (R.I.C.E.).

❖ Elevate the injured limb above the level of the heart.

❖ Use crutches if needed.

❖ Use any over-the-counter non-steroidal anti-inflammatory medication, only if you can tolerate aspirin. In general, this medication should not be used until forty-eight hours after an injury.

DO NOT

❖ Continue your sport.

❖ Put heat on your injured limb.

❖ Use an anti-inflammatory medication immediately.

❖ Strangulate your injured limb with compression.

❖ Elevate the limb by placing your foot on a stool.

❖ Stretch.

❖ Wear shoes that rub on the Achilles tendon.

RED FLAGS

❖ Severe swelling

❖ Severe discoloration

❖ Inability to walk within a few days

❖ Inability to push off when you walk

RETROCALCANEAL BURSITIS

Retrocalcaneal Bursitis is an inflammation of the bursa that lies between your Achilles tendon and heel. This structure is a sac of fluid that allows the Achilles tendon to move in close proximity to the heel without fraying.

This sac can become inflamed with repetitive exercise, increases in frequency, shorter intervals, and longer durations. You will experience pain in the back of your heel, actually right on the back of your heel bone. The pain can be so severe it may require you to cease activity. You may also notice swelling in the heel area. This pain is limited to the heel bone and is usually not as high up as the pain from Achilles tendonitis.

Apply the R.I.C.E principles. Women who wear high-heeled shoes can experience a "pump bump" injury. The heel can rub the area of the retrocalcaneal bursae, causing irritation. Wearing shoes like sandals that do not rub up on the back of the heel can help alleviate this problem.

If pain does not subside in two weeks, consult an orthopaedist. An extra bone in your heel , called a Haglund deformity, sometimes predisposes you to this injury. This extra bone can be surgically removed.

DO

❖ Rest, apply ice and compression, and elevate the limb (R.I.C.E.).
❖ Elevate the injured limb above the level of the heart.
❖ Use crutches if needed.
❖ Try wearing sandals for a period of time.
❖ Use any over-the-counter non-steroidal anti-inflammatory medication, only if you can tolerate aspirin. In general, this medication should not be used until forty-eight hours after an injury.

DO NOT

❖ Continue your sport.
❖ Put heat on your injured limb.
❖ Use an anti-inflammatory medication immediately.
❖ Strangulate your injured limb with compression.
❖ Elevate the limb by placing your foot on a stool.
❖ Wear high-heeled shoes.

RED FLAGS

❖ Severe swelling.
❖ Severe discoloration.
❖ Your bones feel like they move abnormally.
❖ You cannot walk within a few days.

ANKLE SPRAINS

Ankle sprains are injuries to your ankle ligaments and are the most common athletic injury. Sprains result from stretching or tearing your ligaments. Most ankle sprains heal with time and do not require surgical intervention.

You can injure the ligaments on the inside or outside of your ankle. Injury to the outside ankle ligaments is much more common than injury to the inside ankle ligaments.

OUTSIDE (LATERAL) SPRAINS

You can sustain a sprain to the outside or lateral area of your ankle with almost any sporting activity. You can injure any combination of three major ligaments on the lateral (or side) part of your ankle. Such ligaments help to hold your foot bones to your leg bones. When they are intact, they allow these two sets of bones to move normally with respect to each other.

One common way you can sprain your ankle, amongst others, is when you jump up for a shot or rebound during a basketball game and come down on the foot of another player. Your ankle has a tendency to roll inward, and, thus, a sprain can occur.

The position of the foot during the inward roll determines which of the lateral ligaments experiences a sprain. All ligaments can become injured to lesser or greater degrees, no matter what the position of the foot. The force of the injury also determines the nature of ligament injuries.

INSIDE (MEDIAL) SPRAINS

Sprains to the inside or medial area of your ankle have different causes, than lateral ankle sprains. This injury is more commonly seen with football players than with other athletes. The medial ligaments of the ankle hold the tibia, the large bone in the lower leg, to the talus bone in the foot.

Medial ankle sprains often occur when your foot is caught on a playing surface like Astroturf and a force, usually another player hitting your body, causes your tibia, lower leg bone, to rotate inward on the foot. Your foot is essentially facing outward and away from your lower leg bone. This sprain not only affects the ligament of your ankle but, also the ligament between your two lower leg bones as high as the knee. Consequently, you may feel pain all the way up the outside of your lower leg.

There are four degrees of severity for both lateral and medial sprains, from mild to severe. With mild sprains, the ligaments are usually stretched. With severe sprains, the ligaments are generally torn. With sprains in between mild and severe, the ligament can be severely stretched or have partial tears.

When you sprain your ankle you feel pain. You may also hear a pop or hear a tearing sound, depending on the severity of the injury. Your ankle typically becomes swollen and may turn black and blue.

If you sustain a sprained ankle, you should stop the activity and immediately begin to rest, apply ice, use compression, and elevate the limb (the R.I.C.E. principles).

You need rest. Ice will decrease the amount of fluid released and help decrease pain. Compression also helps to decrease swelling. Elevation will help to decrease swelling by reducing the overall blood pressure to the injured area.

If you allow this injury to go untreated, you may see your ankle become black and blue or bruised.

Your ankle sprain may cause you enough pain that you may need crutches. If you have a significant amount of swelling, have an x-ray taken to rule out a fracture.

Most ankle sprains will heal by themselves with the treatment I have recommended. If you have a mild to intermediate type sprain, immobilization with the gradual commencement of stretching and strengthening exercises may help you return to sports more quickly. However, if you have a severe ankle sprain and are quite athletic, you may need surgery to repair torn ligaments.

DO

❖ Rest, apply ice and compression and elevate the limb (R.I.C.E.).

❖ Use crutches, if necessary.

❖ Elevate your injured limb above the level of your heart.

❖ Use any over-the-counter non-steroidal anti-inflammatory medication, only if you can tolerate aspirin. In general, this medication should not be used until forty-eight hours after an injury.

DO NOT

❖ Continue your sport.

❖ Put heat on your injured limb.

❖ Use an anti-inflammatory medication immediately.

❖ Strangulate your injured limb with compression.

❖ Elevate the limb by placing your foot on a stool.

❖ Stretch.

Red Flags

❖ Severe swelling.

❖ Severe dislocation.

❖ Abnormal movement of bones.

❖ Inability to walk within a few days.

THE FOOT

Read this section if your pain and swelling are located lower than your ankle. You can sustain injuries to your mid-foot (Lis Franc sprains, as well as fractures), the bottom of your foot (plantar fasciitis), the nerves on the inside of your foot and ankle (tarsal tunnel syndrome), or your big toe (turf toe sprains).

FOOT FRACTURES

STRESS FRACTURES (MID-FOOT INJURIES)

Your foot experiences great force during walking and running. During the evolutionary process, we developed from animals that walked on all fours (quadrupeds) to animals that walked with a two-legged gait (bipeds). Our feet underwent changes to compensate for these great forces. The present bony, ligamentous, muscular, and joint structures of the foot permit us to use bipedal movement without injury.

However, as with other parts of the body, on occasion, the foot bones can become fatigued. Bones in the foot can sustain stress fractures as a result of repetitive, chronic, intense forces experienced during running, jumping, and other athletic endeavors.

The bones that most commonly experience stress fractures are the metatarsals. These bones are located about half-way between your heel and your toes. A stress fracture occurs not because of a single blow but because of many intense blows or stress loads.

However, the sudden pain is actually a final symptom in a long process. You had probably already fatigued your bone to the point that when you finally placed stress on it your bone broke with minimal loading.

Up to the point it broke, your foot bone was probably bending abnormally. This condition can be compared to a branch of a tree. When you bend a tree branch, it bends. At some point, however, you can break the branch.

Pain from a stress fracture can be severe, but this is not always the case. The pain is also usually limited to the bone that is broken. The pain will usually require you to cease activity. You may even feel like the bones within your foot move when you walk. You may also have a small amount of swelling.

If you suspect you have a stress fracture in your foot, begin R.I.C.E. You may need crutches. You should also obtain an x-ray of your foot. Initial x-rays can sometimes be negative. A break may not appear on an x-ray for up to two weeks. Therefore, do not be surprised if your physician orders a bone-scan.

The definitive treatment for a stress fracture is immobilization, perhaps even a cast. Consult an orthopaedist regarding the treatment of your injury. Some fractures may not heal and eventually require surgery.

DO

* Rest, apply ice, use compression, and elevate the limb (R.I.C.E.).
* Elevate the injured limb above the level of the heart.
* Use crutches, if needed.
* Use any over-the-counter non-steroidal anti-inflammatory medication, only if you can tolerate aspirin. In general, this medication should not be used until forty-eight hours after an injury.

DO NOT

* Continue your sport.
* Put heat on your injured limb.
* Use an anti-inflammatory medication immediately.
* Strangulate your injured limb with compression.
* Elevate the limb by placing your foot on a stool.
* Stretch.

RED FLAGS

* Severe swelling.
* Severe discoloration.
* Your bones feel like they move abnormally.
* You cannot walk within a few days.

FOOT INFLAMMATION

Inflammation can occur in the bottom part of your foot (the plantar fasciitis tissues) or to the nerves surrounding your ankle and foot (Tarsal Tunnel Syndrome).

PLANTAR FASCIITIS
(INJURIES TO THE BOTTOM OF THE FEET)

Plantar fasciitis is an inflammation of the tissues (fascia) on the bottom of your feet (plantar), not on your skin. This injury can occur in almost any sporting event that requires using your feet for long periods of time. However, the injury can occur simply from walking. Athletes with cavus feet, or high arches, are especially susceptible to this injury.

The plantar fascia runs from your heel to your toes. The tissue acts like a windlass on a boat. As you bend your toes upward, the plantar fascia tries to wind up. By doing so, it pulls on your heel and gives your foot stability for propulsion.

Plantar fascia can cause burning or pain on the undersurface of your heel and foot, primarily on the inside. This pain is often more severe in the morning and is reduced with walking and other activities. You may notice it is severe after sitting for long periods of time.

The pain can be quite disabling. You may also find yourself unable to participate in sports after a long warm-up.

Stretching and strengthening the fascia, ligaments, and muscles in both the fronts and backs of your feet will help decrease some of the pain. Prior to walking or exercising, you may want to soak your feet in a warm bath. Warming will help loosen the structures in your feet. After walking and exercising, you may want to apply ice to your feet to help decrease some of the inflammation and swelling.

Plantar fasciitis can take up to several months to heal. You may have recurrences even after you think you are healing. In general, a thorough stretching routine will help to alleviate the symptoms over a period of time.

If you are concerned about pain or burning that does not diminish after six weeks, consult an orthopaedist. Surgery is almost never indicated. However, a physician can recommend proper stretching and strengthening exercises. Anti-inflammatory medication may also help.

DO

❖ Rest, apply ice, use compression, and elevate the limb (R.I.C.E.).

❖ Elevate the injured limb above the level of the heart.

❖ Use crutches, if needed.

❖ Heat and message the limb prior to exercise.

❖ Strengthen the muscles in front of your leg.

❖ Use any over-the-counter non-steroidal anti-inflammatory medication, only if you can tolerate aspirin. In general, this medication should not be used until forty-eight hours after an injury.

DO NOT

❖ Continue your sport.

❖ Put heat on your injured limb after exercise.

❖ Apply ice before exercise.

❖ Use an anti-inflammatory medication immediately.

❖ Wear floppy or inappropriate shoes.

RED FLAGS

❖ Severe swelling.

❖ Severe discoloration.

❖ Your bones feel like they move abnormally.

❖ You cannot walk within a few days.

NEURITIS
(INJURY TO THE NERVE ON THE INSIDE OF YOUR FOOT)

Tarsal tunnel syndrome is an injury that is an inflammation of a nerve or a neuritis. Like carpal tunnel syndrome, this injury can result from compression of a nerve. The tibial nerve in your foot is located on the inside of your ankle. This nerve can become compressed along its path into your foot. Such a compression can be caused by tight ligaments, fascia, or muscles, as well as by extra bones or a ganglion.

This syndrome can result from repetitive use or from an anatomical abnormality, such as an extra bone. Furthermore, it can mimic the signs and symptoms of plantar fasciitis. You may experience pain or burning along various parts of your feet and toes. If the nerve injury is severe, you may also experience weakness in the muscles of your feet.

You can usually locate the nerve by gently tapping on it as it courses around the inside of your ankle. When you do, you may experience a shock-like sensation in your foot and toes. When a nerve becomes irritated, known as neuritis, it becomes hypersensitive. Tapping on the tibial nerve does not normally cause shocks. When it is irritated, however, it is hypersensitive so such shocks are common.

Consult an orthopaedist regarding this injury. The doctor likely will usually treat tarsal tunnel syndrome surgically, if the signs and symptoms warrant. Avoid any self-treatment for this injury.

Be aware that numbness, tingling, or weakness of your foot may be caused by a back problem. If you have back pain in conjunction with these signs and symptoms of foot injuries, consult an orthopaedist.

DO

❖ Rest, apply ice, use compression, and elevate the limb (R.I.C.E.).

❖ Elevate the injured limb above the level of the heart.

❖ Use crutches, if needed.

❖ Use any over-the-counter non-steroidal anti-inflammatory medication, only if you can tolerate aspirin. In general, this medication should not be used until forty-eight hours after an injury.

DO NOT

❖ Continue your sport.

❖ Put heat on your injured limb.

❖ Use an anti-inflammatory medication immediately.

❖ Strangulate your injured limb with compression.

❖ Elevate your foot by placing it on a footstool.

RED FLAGS

❖ Severe swelling.

❖ Severe discoloration.

❖ Your bones feel like they move abnormally.

❖ You cannot walk within a few days.

❖ Severe numbness or tingling in your foot.

FOOT SPRAINS

TURF TOE SPRAINS (BIG TOE INJURIES)

Turf toe injuries occurs when athletes, attempting to stop running quickly, find their great toe bends upwards beyond its normal motion. Turf toe injury is most commonly experienced by football players who play on a hard playing surface like Astroturf.

Turf toe is not limited to football players. Those playing basketball, racquetball, and volleyball can experience this injury, as can athletes in any sport requiring them to stop and start quickly.

The great toe contains the big knuckle or metatarsophalangeal joint (MTP) where the injury occurs. You may immediately experience pain on the bottom and sides of your great toe at the big knuckle. The degree of injury varies between mild and severe. This injury is a combination of a strain to your tendons, a sprain to your ligaments, and MTP subluxation or dislocation in which the two bones abnormally move away from each other.

If you experience a mild injury, you may still be able to continue to participate in your sporting event. Wearing a shoe with a sturdy toe-box will usually allow you to play. This type of shoe prevents your great toe from bending upwards, which causes great pain.

If your injury is severe, you may not be able to play even with a sturdy shoe. Your injured toe may also need a form of immobilization, perhaps even a cast, until the severely stretched or torn structures heal. This injury occasionally requires surgery.

If you sustain a turf toe injury, immobilize your foot and refrain from exercise. If the injury does not heal within two weeks, consult an orthopaedist.

DO

❖ Rest, apply ice, use compression, and elevate the limb above the level of the heart (R.I.C.E.).

❖ Wear a shoe with a sturdy toe-box.

❖ Use any over-the-counter non-steroidal anti-inflammatory medication, only if you can tolerate aspirin. In general, this medication should not be used until forty-eight hours after an injury.

DO NOT

❖ Continue your sport.

❖ Put heat on your injured limb.

❖ Use an anti-inflammatory medication immediately.

❖ Strangulate your injured limb with compression.

❖ Elevate the limb by placing your foot on a stool.

❖ Wear floppy or inappropriate shoes.

RED FLAGS

❖ Severe swelling.

* Severe discoloration.
* Your bones feel like they move abnormally.
* You cannot walk within a few days.

LIS FRANC SPRAINS (MID-FOOT INJURIES)

Lis Franc was a surgeon in Napoleon's army. During the mobilization of the French troops, the militia would ride horseback. They were often injured after being thrown from their saddles when their horses became startled by the sound of cannons firing. On occasion, the rider's foot would become caught in the stirrup, breaking the foot halfway back to the heel.

Lis Franc was thus compelled to amputate these injured feet through the mid-foot area. Thus, the MTP joints located half-way between the toes and the heel were later called the Lis Franc joint.

A Lis Franc injury can be a sprain of your foot's ligaments or a dislocation or fracture of your foot bones. You may experience the immediate onset of pain with this injury and need to cease activities. The pain will be limited to the area halfway between your heel and the tip of your toes. You may, in addition, feel like the bones in the mid-portion of your foot are not in the right place.

If you think you have sustained such an injury, begin R.I.C.E. Use crutches to reduce the load on your foot. A splint may also help relieve the pain.

You should seek the opinion of an orthopaedist. X-rays, especially stress x-rays, may be needed to make a diagnosis.

DO

* Rest, apply ice, use compression, and elevate the limb (R.I.C.E.).
* Elevate the injured limb above the level of the heart.
* Wear a sturdy shoe.
* Use crutches, if needed.
* Use any over-the-counter non-steroidal anti-

inflammatory medication, only if you can tolerate aspirin. In general, this medication should not be used until forty-eight hours after an injury.

DO NOT

❖ Continue your sport.

❖ Put heat on your injured limb.

❖ Use an anti-inflammatory medication immediately.

❖ Strangulate your injured limb with compression.

❖ Elevate the limb by placing your foot on a stool.

❖ Wear floppy or inappropriate shoes.

RED FLAGS

❖ Severe swelling.

❖ Severe discoloration.

❖ Your bones feel like they move abnormally.

❖ You cannot walk within a few days.

CHAPTER 16:

THE LOWER LEG AND KNEE

Injuries to your lower leg and knee are common among athletes. Lower leg injuries include those to the tibia, or large bone, or to the fibula, the smaller bone, as well as to muscles and fascia. Knee injuries include those to the cartilage, ligaments, or tendons of the knee joint.

LOWER LEG

COMPARTMENT SYNDROME

Compartment syndromes, like shin splints, can occur with repetitive use. However, compartment syndromes are not as common as shin splints.

The muscles in your lower leg are connected to the bone by fascia. Certain groups of muscles are enclosed in sheaths of fascia called compartments. Four major compartments occur in your leg. The superficial and the deep are behind the leg. The lateral and anterior are on the outside and front of your leg.

During exercise, your leg muscles undergo repetitive contractions that cause increased blood flow. This increases the size of your muscles. If you exercise regularly, the size of your muscles can increase, you can have abnormal muscle enlargement, or hypertrophy.

When a muscle increases in size by either increased blood flow or hypertrophy, the fascial sheaths surrounding the muscles sometimes do not expand. The size of the compartment does not increase its volume, even though the muscle is trying to do so.

Within these compartments are nerves, as well as arteries that supply blood to the tissues. When your muscle increases in size but cannot expand because of fascial restraints or compartments, the nerves, arteries, and muscles themselves can become compressed. This is known as compartment syndrome.

If you were to fill a waterbed too full of water, at some point the plastic would resist the water. If there were objects inside your waterbed, they might become crushed, depending, of course, on the force with which the water was being propelled into the waterbed. It might burst at any time.

This is what happens when one experiences a compartment syndrome. When muscles have no room to expand, they press against the fascial sheaths like the water might press against the plastic of a waterbed.

Tissues in compartments become compressed with exercise. If you develop this injury, you may experience pain, numbness, or tingling in your legs. The pain can be similar to that experienced with shin splints. However, because of the four compartments in your leg, pain can be experienced in any part of the leg.

The initial problem you may experience is pain or burning anywhere in your leg. When you begin to exercise, the pain is usually mild, but it increases with duration and ceases with rest. If you feel pain that is not along the inside of your leg, you probably have a compartment syndrome, not a shin splint. This is not, however, always the case.

With a severe compartment syndrome, your leg and foot muscles may not function. You may have difficulty lifting your toes or ankles. You may not be able to push off when walking. The weakness, loss of function, and numbness or tingling typically occur later in the process.

Compartment syndrome usually occurs after long durations of exercise. The injury is not often seen when someone is beginning to perform an exercise for the first time.

Stretch before and after exercise to prevent this injury. Use heat before you stretch and exercise, and ice after you exercise and stretch to reduce the likelihood of this injury. You can still sustain this injury, however, despite a thorough stretching.

DO

* ❖ Stretch prior to exercise.
* ❖ Elevate your leg.
* ❖ Apply ice to your leg.
* ❖ Immediately seek medical attention.

DO NOT

* ❖ Use heat on your injury.
* ❖ Delay seeking medical attention.
* ❖ Continue participation.
* ❖ Use an anti-inflammatory medication.

Seek medical attention as soon as possible for this injury, preferably from an orthopaedist with sports medicine training. If you experience a loss of muscle function, numbness, or tingling immediately during or just after exercise, cease exercising and elevate the leg. Icing may help the pain, but avoid prolonged icing, as well as heating.

FRACTURES

STRESS FRACTURES

Stress fractures can also occur to the tibia or lower leg bone. This type of injury is less common than shin splints and compartment syndromes. Such fractures typically occur with activities like running and aerobics that repeatedly require the body to leave the ground and return to it.

A stress fracture is a break in a bone. The break occurs because of repetitive cycling of the bone that causes the bone to become fatigued and break.

A lower leg stress fracture differs from the fracture that occurs as a result of a blow or fall. With stress fractures, the breaks are usually non-displaced. That is, the ends of the bones that break do not become out of alignment.

These fractures sometimes affect only a portion of the bone and are not complete fractures through the entire width of the bone. Such fractures can occur in the leg bone, as well as in the bones of the feet.

When you experience a stress fracture, you will feel an immediate onset of pain on the inside or outside of your leg, ankle, knee, or foot. The pain is usually quite uncomfortable.

You may sometimes not feel the pain until you have stopped exercising. With such fractures, you usually will not have any numbness, tingling, or loss of function. You may not see large amounts of swelling.

The pain can be quite similar to that which results from shin splints. Thus, you may find it difficult to differentiate between the two injuries.

Stretching prior to exercise probably will not prevent this injury. Because this is an uncommon injury, if you experience pain in your leg without a loss of function, numbness, or tingling, you probably have a shin splint. The use of properly cushioned running shoes, will help to prevent this injury.

If you suspect you have a stress fracture, the self-treatment I recommend is to stop exercising, apply ice to the injury, administer a splint, and use crutches.

DO

- ❖ Wear a cushioned running shoe.
- ❖ Use crutches.
- ❖ Seek medical attention.
- ❖ Apply ice after the injury.
- ❖ Have an x-ray taken.

❖ Splint your injury.

DO NOT
❖ Continue participation.
❖ Use heat on your injury.
❖ Delay seeking medical attention.

If your pain does not diminish in two weeks, consult a doctor. An x-ray can typically help a doctor determine whether you have this injury. If you have an x-ray at the first sign of pain, the injury may not appear on the x-ray. Bone scans are occasionally used to help make the diagnosis since the fracture is sometimes not visible with x-rays.

An orthopaedist should treat this injury that may require some type of immobilization, perhaps a cast.

RED FLAGS
❖ Severe pain.
❖ Inability to walk.
❖ You hear your bones crack.

TIBIA FRACTURES
You can also sustain a fracture to your tibia, the lower leg bone. The cause of the injury is usually a direct blow.

However, a tibia fracture can also be a stress fracture that occurs over a period of time and results from repeated stress loads.

Advice regarding what you should do and not do for a tibia fracture, as well as the red flags, are the same as that for a stress fracture. Consult an orthopaedist.

POPLITEAL ARTERY SYNDROME
This is an uncommon injury. With hypertrophy or abnormal enlargement of the muscles around the back of your knee, you may begin to experience a dull aching pain in your lower leg. These muscles may also feel weak.

Fascial bands of tissue surround the popliteal artery located behind your knee. When these bands become tightened because of enlarged muscles in this area, they can squeeze the artery.

This popliteal artery supplies blood to all the tissues of your lower leg. When constriction diminishes the blood supply, the lower leg may ache or feel weak.

Rest should eliminate your symptoms. Applying ice or heat will probably not be beneficial. If the pain and aching do not diminish in a few weeks, consult your doctor.

SUPERFICIAL PERONEAL NERVE ENTRAPMENT SYNDROME

This injury can mimic a compartment syndrome. Some physicians suspect it is caused by a compartment syndrome.

The superficial peroneal nerve exits a fascial sheath along the outside of the lower third of your leg. A fascial band can cause constriction of the nerve as it passes out from under the sheath to run just below your skin.

The peroneal nerve supplies sensation to the lower and outside portion of your ankle and leg. If this nerve becomes compressed, you may experience pain or numbness. This injury is considered a compression of the nerve.

TISSUE INFLAMMATION AND COMPRESSION

SHIN SPLINTS

Shin splints, also called medial tibial syndrome (MTS), is a common injury to the lower legs. The injury frequently occurs when you are new to an exercise. It also occurs when you are a veteran of the sport who decides to increase either the interval, resistance, duration, or frequency of your exercise. The repetitive nature of exercise can predispose you to this type of injury.

Fascia attach the muscles on the inner and outer part of your leg to the leg bone, or tibia. The fascia is inserted into the periosteum, the outer coating of your tibia bone. As you exercise, this area is subjected to stress caused by muscle contractions.

With repetitive contractions, this area can become inflamed as a healing response. Small tears in the fascia can occur. When the tissue becomes inflamed, it gives off such substances as bradykinins and substance "P". They interact with your leg's nerves and stimulate the nerves that go to your brain. Your brain recognizes this stimulation as pain or burning.

During exercise and with an increase in the intensity of your exercise, you may feel a burning sensation along the inner part of your shin. This burning can be so severe that you must cease your exercise. In addition, once you have noticed this discomfort, your attempt to return to exercise, even the following day, can cause you the same pain.

This pain may not diminish when you stop exercising. You may experience this pain during walking and even while simply moving your ankle up and down while seated.

Shin splint pain generally occurs along a line from your big toe to the inner side of your kneecap. If you experience pain at the extremes of this line, either near your ankle or kneecap, it is probably not due to shin splints.

You can take several measures to avoid this injury. Stretching thoroughly prior to athletic participation can decrease the incidence of shin splints. Stretching will loosen up the muscles, tendons, and fascia of your legs, thereby decreasing the likelihood of tearing these structures.

Stretch both the muscles in back of your leg and in front of your leg, the ankle, and toe extensors. A stretching text or athletic trainer can instruct you on how to stretch these muscles.

If you are predisposed to shin splints or have had this injury in the past, consider using a heating pack or warm soaks prior to exercise. Avoid applying ice prior to exercising. This simply tightens up your muscles and makes you less flexible. Wrap heating packs in a towel, and place them around your leg. Place the heat directly along the line from your great toe to the inner part of your kneecap.

If you experience shin splints despite stretching and following the equipment instructions, you may experience great amounts of discomfort and disability. You will want to return to exercising as soon as possible. If this injury is your only injury, it will heal.

You can use several techniques to decrease the pain and return to exercising. You have injured the tissues on the inside of your leg, so there may be small amounts of swelling. The tissue has been torn slightly. Thus, the capillaries, the tissues that carry fluid in this region, may allow fluid out of their channels.

During the first twenty-four to forty-eight hours, avoid heating packs and warm soaks, even though the warmth may feel good. Heating causes increased fluid to accumulate in the injured area, which causes further swelling.

Use ice packs to decrease the pain caused by the fluid that the capillaries are releasing. Wrap ice packs in a towel and place them on the area that hurts. Avoid directly exposing the skin to cold.

Ice achieves two goals. If it is left on long enough, the affected area begins to become numb. An anesthetic affect will then occur, decreasing your pain.

Apply ice for twenty-four to forty-eight hours. Administer it for a length of twenty minutes every four hours, or intermittently, for as often as necessary until you feel some pain relief. Then begin stretching out the muscles in the front and back of your leg. Do this quite slowly at first and only up the point at which you experience mild discomfort. You want to avoid retearing the tissue.

After the initial injury, your body's tissues will be inflamed. Use ice to control the inflammation until it has subsided. Your body will then try to repair the injured tissues. During the healing process, your injured leg will feel tight, which is normal. Avoid trying to heal too fast to avoid reinjuring the healing tissue.

DO

❖ Stretch and warm up prior to exercise.

❖ Use heat prior to exercise.

❖ Massage your limb prior to exercise.

❖ Use a cushioned training shoe.

❖ Use ice after exercise.

❖ Use an anti-inflammatory medication after the first twenty-four to forty-eight hours.

❖ An anti-inflammatory medication should be taken on a full stomach and only if you can safely take aspirin.

You will generally need to wait two weeks after sustaining this injury until you return to activities. The usual length of time for complete healing can be as long as six weeks.

When you are returning to activities, stretch prior to exercise. If you cannot move your ankle like you did before the injury, you probably should not be returning to strenuous activities. Go slowly, stretch, and use heat prior to exercise after the pain has subsided.

DO NOT

❖ Continue participation.

❖ Take an anti-inflammatory medication within the first twenty-four to forty-eight hours.

❖ Use heat after exercise.

❖ Apply ice prior to exercise.

If, after two weeks of resting without exercise, you still have pain, consult a doctor.

RED FLAGS

❖ No pain relief after two weeks.

❖ Numbness or tingling.

❖ Loss of function of your foot, leg or toes.

Other injuries can mimic a shin splint. These include

compartment syndromes, popliteal artery syndrome, super-ficial peroneal nerve entrapment, and stress fractures. These injuries can be more disabling, so you should consult a physician.

KNEE

A knee dislocation is an orthopaedic emergency. You should immediately seek medical attention from an orthopaedist. This injury is the result of significant trauma. Football players, gymnasts, and other athletes who exper-ience great direct force to the knee can incur this injury.

If you dislocate your kneecap, you may feel it is a knee dislocation. However, a kneecap dislocation is not as severe an injury as a dislocation of the knee.

Using ice after activity may help. Warming up thoroughly and stretching your kneecap may help decrease the pain or dislocation.

Your doctor can show you mobilizing techniques to prevent the recurrence of this injury. Some braces and taping methods may also help.

LIGAMENT SPRAINS AND TEARS

Four major ligaments surround your knee joint. The anterior cruciate ligament (ACL) and posterior cruciate ligament (PCL) are inside the joint and the medial collateral liagment (MCL) and the lateral collateral liagment (LCL) are outside the joint.

ANTERIOR CRUCIATE LIGAMENTS (ACL) AND POSTERIOR CRUCIATE LIGAMENTS (PCL)

You might have heard of injuries to these ligaments in professional football players. Cruciate ligaments, sometimes referred to as the "crucial" ligaments, cross inside your knee. They closcly resemble an "X" and allow your knee to function normally during daily activity.

Two ligaments support your knee on the outside of the

joint. The medial collateral ligament (MLC) is on the inner part of your knee. The lateral collateral ligament (LCL) is on the outer part.

Most of the injuries that occur to the ACL are the result of an acute injury. You might have received a blow or a fall, or have been involved in a motor vehicle accident.

ACL injuries can occur when you ski, play football or basketball, or catch your leg in a rut.

If you are skiing and catch an inside edge and fall to the opposite side, your ski continues on its edge and moves away from your body. This can injure your ACL. Even the best of skiers can sustain this injury.

ACL injuries are usually tears that can range from minor to major. Some may heal, and others may require surgery. If you tear one of the ligaments on the inside of your knee, you may hear a pop. Your knee may then swell and become painful. However, the pain commonly diminishes within twenty-four to forty-eight hours.

If you do not receive treatment, your knee will generally swell to the size of a grapefruit. In addition, when you later walk on uneven ground or when you plant your feet and turn when running your knee may feel unstable, as if it wants to give out.

Injuries to the posterior cruciate ligament usually occur from a direct blow to the knee or the thigh bone. PCL injuries are more common with motorvehicle accidents, especially if you throw your knees up on the dashboard in a crash. Your knee will swell. You may also experience pain that may diminish within twenty-four to forty-eight hours.

FOR ACL AND PCL, DO

❖ Rest.
❖ Apply ice.
❖ Elevate the limb.
❖ Use crutches.
❖ Seek medical attention.
❖ Use a brace.

For ACL And PCL, DO NOT

❖   Continue with cutting activities.

❖   Use heat.

❖   Use an anti-inflammatory medication.

For ACL And PCL, Red Flags

❖   Your knee swells the size of a grapefruit.

❖   Your knee gives out.

❖   You hear a pop.

Medial And Lateral Collateral Ligaments (MLC/LCL)

Injuries to the ligament on the inner side, the medial collateral ligament (MCL), are more common than injuries to the lateral collateral ligament (LCL) on the outside of your knee.

Forces that push your knee inward or toward the other knee will cause injury to the MCL. Forces that push your leg outward can cause injury to the LCL. With any injury, you can tear more than one ligament.

With both MCL and LCL injuries, your knee will swell. The swelling will not be as large as it would with an injury to one of your cruciate ligaments. You will have pain, and you may hear a pop. You may also have a feeling of instability when you walk. Some of these injuries will heal by themselves, but some will require surgery.

If you suspect you have injured one of these ligaments, use ice and elevate your leg. Stop participating in your activity. Unlike tendonitis, which may occur over time, these injuries occur with a single event.

Consult an orthopaedist for such injuries.

For MCL And LCL Injuries, DO

❖   Rest.

❖   Apply ice.

❖   Elevate the limb.

❖   Use crutches.

❖ Use a brace.

❖ Seek medical attention.

For MCL And LCL Injuries, DO NOT

❖ Continue with activity.

❖ Use heat.

❖ Stretch.

For MCL And LCL Injuries, Red Flags

❖ Your knee swells the size of a grapefruit.

❖ Your knee gives out.

Meniscal Injuries

The lateral and medial menisci are half-moon shaped bodies of cartilage in your knee joint. They serve as shock absorbers. This cartilage is slightly different than the cartilage on the ends of your bones. When you twist your knee, these structures can be torn. They can also be injured when you injure your knee ligaments.

If you injure one of these menisci, you will feel knee pain and your knee may swell slightly. You may even notice you feel a click or a catching sensation in your knee when you walk. If the tear is large, your knee may lock into position.

With this injury, apply ice, elevate your knee, and cease activities.

DO

❖ Rest.

❖ Apply ice.

❖ Elevate the limb.

DO NOT

❖ Continue with activity.

❖ Use heat.

Red Flags

❖ Your knee locks into position.

❖ Your knee catches when you walk.

Consult an orthopaedist. Small tears will sometimes heal themselves, but larger, more complex tears may require arthroscopic surgery.

TISSUE INFLAMMATION

TENDONITIS OF THE ILIOTIBIAL BAND AND PES ANSERINUS

Inflammation of tendons, or tendonitis, around your knee can cause knee pain. The pain usually results from repetitive motions and not from acute injuries. If you suddenly sustain an injury to your knee, you probably do not have tendonitis.

Two major groups of tendons around your knee can become inflamed. One group is the pes anserinus on the inside of your knee. The other is the iliotibial band (ITB) on the outside of your knee.

If you are an active runner, especially one who runs on uneven ground, you may develop an inflammation of these tendons. Inflammation of the tendon on the inside of your leg can result from tendonitis of the pes anserinus. You will feel pain below and near the inner side of your kneecap.

However, this pain can also be caused by bursitis in this area. Both bursitis and tendonitis are usually caused by repeatedly performing the same activities.

The pain can also be caused by meniscal and ligamentous injuries, though such injuries are caused by a sudden event. Inflammation of the tendon on the outside of your leg can result from tendonitis of the ITB. This pain is typically felt below and near the outer side of your kneecap. Your ITB can snap around your kneecap as you walk, causing you pain.

However, pain on the outside of your knee can also be attributed to problems with the movement of your kneecap.

DO

* ❖ Cease activity.
* ❖ Apply ice.
* ❖ Stretch.

❖ Use any over-the-counter non-steroidal anti-inflammatory medication, only if you can tolerate aspirin. This drug can be taken for tendonitis and bursitis In general, this medication should not be used until forty-eight hours after an injury.

If you think you have knee tendonitis, stop performing your activity to see if the pain diminishes. Applying ice immediately after experiencing pain for twenty-four to forty-eight hours can help. Stretching can also aid in preventing a recurrence.

DO NOT

❖ Apply heat after experiencing pain.
❖ Continue with your activity.

Try to stretch the muscles on the inside of your leg by performing split-like maneuvers. Stretch those on the outside of your leg by moving your leg downwards over the edge of a sofa while lying on your side. Refer to any stretching text that tells you how to stretch the tensor fascia lata and the pes anserinus tendons.

RED FLAGS

❖ Inability to walk.
❖ Your knee balloons to the size of a grapefruit.
❖ You heard a loud snap.

KNEECAP IRRITATION
(PATELLAR RETINACULAR INFLAMMATION)

Pain on the outside of your knee can also be due to inflammation of the patellar retinaculum. This structure connects your kneecap to the outside musculature of your leg.

Your kneecap may occasionally move in the wrong direction. This is called patellar maltracking. When this occurs, you can repeatedly feel tension on the outer side of your kneecap. The patellar retinaculum on the outside of your knee can become inflamed causing debilitating pain.

You will often feel pain on the front and outer part of your kneecap. The tissue on the outside of your kneecap may also be tender to touch. In fact, if you move your kneecap from side to side, you may feel pain.

DO

❖ Rest.
❖ Stretch both front and back thigh muscles.
❖ Mobilize your kneecap.
❖ Strengthen your inner thigh muscles.

If you experience patellar retinacular inflammation, you should rest, and apply ice. Avoid walking up stairs or crossing your legs, both of which place pressure on your kneecap that causes pain.

Mobilize your patella by grasping your kneecap, despite tenderness, and moving it side to side and up and down and rotate it around in a circular motion as far as possible. Move it both clockwise and counterclockwise.

You will need to strengthen the muscles on the inside of your kneecap to prevent this pain from recurring.

DO NOT

❖ Use stairs.
❖ Sit with your legs crossed.
❖ Perform pounding activities.

RED FLAGS

❖ Your knee balloons up.
❖ Your kneecap jumps.
❖ You cannot walk.

CHONDROMALACIA OR SICK CARTILAGE

Articular cartilage attaches to the ends of your bones, as well as to the undersurface of your patella. This cartilage acts as a shock absorber by ensuring a fluid gliding motion to your knee joint.

This cartilage can become injured when you bang your knee or injure a ligament. If you stretch or tear a ligament, your knee joint may not function properly. When this happens, cartilage wear can occur.

The cartilage then begins to deteriorate and become inflamed. The degree of wear determines the degree of cartilage deterioration. Chondromalacia is the medical term for cartilage deterioration and inflammation.

During the course of this process, you may experience pain. Whether it comes from related synovitis or from chondromalacia is not important.

You usually feel more pain in your knee in the morning and after you have been still for a period of time. Your knee may also feel stiff. With movement, your knee may warm up, and cause the pain to diminish somewhat.

Activities like walking up and down stairs and sitting with your legs crossed may aggravate the pain. Your knee may also swell intermittently. The amount of swelling, however, may be small.

DO

* Rest.
* Use ice.
* Avoid stairs.
* Avoid sitting with your legs crossed.
* Use any over-the-counter non-steroidal anti-inflammatory medication, only if you can tolerate aspirin. In general, this medication should not be used until forty-eight hours after an injury.

DO NOT

❖ Continue with high impact activity.

❖ Use heat.

Fractures of the Kneecap

Fractures of the kneecap usually result from a direct blow to the knee. Vigorous jumping can also cause the bone to fracture. More often, though, injuries from jumping tear the tendon that goes from your kneecap to your lower leg bone.

If you sustain an injury to your kneecap that leads to a fracture, your knee will swell markedly. Your knee can commonly swell at least to the size of a grapefruit. The skin will also be quite black and blue.

You may also be unable to straighten your leg because the fracture has torn some of the surrounding tissues. The pain will be severe.

DO

❖ Rest, apply ice and compression, and elevate the injury (R.I.C.E.).

❖ Use a splint.

❖ Use crutches.

❖ Consult a doctor.

DO NOT

❖ Use an anti-inflammatory medication.

❖ Continue to walk.

❖ Apply heat.

If you have this injury, you will need to have an x-ray. Consult an orthopaedic surgeon regarding this injury.

Cartilage or Bone (Osteochondral) Lesions

Articular cartilage covers the ends of your bone. The cartilage bonds to the bone. Acute injuries to your knee joint can shear off portions of the cartilage and bone complex.

The result can be a loose body in your joint. You may sense pain or the feeling that something is actually floating around in your knee. Your knee may also catch or lock so that you cannot move it.

You may need arthroscopic surgery to remove the floating piece. Consult your doctor if your symptoms and signs do not disappear within two weeks.

DISLOCATIONS (SUBLUXATIONS)

The Kneecap

Your kneecap can also dislocate or track abnormally. You may then experience pain in different areas of your kneecap during different activities. This injury may also cause wear to the cartilage found on the undersurface of your kneecap.

When you dislocate your kneecap, you feel a twisting type force to your kneecap that makes it feel like it popped out of its socket.

Your knee may swell and your kneecap may pop. When this happens, you may have pain on both the inner and outer parts of your kneecap. When you dislocate your kneecap, you can sometimes knock off a piece of cartilage.

DO

* ❖ Rest.
* ❖ Apply ice.
* ❖ Elevate the injured limb.
* ❖ Strengthen the muscles on the inner thigh.
* ❖ Wear a kneecap brace.

DO NOT

* ❖ Use heat.
* ❖ Continue with the same activity.

RED FLAGS

* ❖ Your kneecap remains dislocated.
* ❖ Your kneecap feels like it will pop out of its socket when you walk.

CHAPTER 17:

THE THIGH AND HIP

—— • —— • —— • —— • ——

THE THIGH

CONTUSIONS (BRUISES)

Contusions or bruises of the thigh usually occur from a direct blow. This injury commonly occurs in football players. The cause of injury is usually a helmet to the thigh.

You will experience acute pain that may be so severe you cannot walk normally. In addition, there may be swelling of the thigh muscles. Resting and applying ice can help. The gradual institution of stretching exercises can also help.

MYOSITIS OSSIFICANS (MUSCLE KNOT) AND HETEROTOPIC OSSIFICATION (BONE KNOT)

You might develop a knot at the area of thigh trauma, depending on the force, as well as the amount of muscle you injure. Myositis ossificans (MO) is a thigh muscle knot that may feel like a bone.

A heterotopic ossification (HO) is a thigh bone knot that occurs through a similar process. Trauma occurred to your thigh bone. Both injuries may heal with time.

The extent of MO or HO injury determines the degree of your pain with motion. Surgery is occasionally required to remove the mass.

DO

* ❖ Rest.
* ❖ Apply ice.

DO NOT

* ❖ Apply heat.
* ❖ Continue with activity.
* ❖ Have the lesion drained.

RED FLAGS

* ❖ You find a knot that has arisen without a direct blow.

STRAINS

Injuries that occur to the thigh and hip are usually strains of the muscles in the front, back, and inner part of the thigh.

The muscles in front of your leg include the quadriceps and the sartorius muscle. The quadriceps consists of four muscles: the vastus lateralis, the vastus medialis, the vastus intermedius, and the rectus femoris. All four muscles are joined at your knee creating one tendon in your kneecap, the patella. This tendon continues past your patella and inserts on your lower leg bone, the tibia.

The hamstring muscles are in back of your leg. They consist of the biceps femoris, the long and short head, the semimembranosus, and the semitendinosus.

Finally, the adductor group of muscles on the inside of your leg includes the pectineus, gracilis, adductor magnus, adductor longus, and adductor brevis.

TYPES OF INJURIES

HIP POINTERS

The term "hip pointer" is often used by athletic trainers working with football players. The term is a misnomer since the injury has nothing to do with your hip.

Hip pointers are strains of the muscle, usually the quadriceps in front of your leg. They usually occur at the place the muscles insert into your pelvis bone and can be quite painful.

A hip pointer is usually the result of an acute injury. If you sustain this injury, you will feel pain where the muscle inserts. When you place your hands on your hips, you can feel a ridge of bone. This is the area hip pointers generally occur.

If you sustain this injury, rest and apply ice to the tender area. This is a strain type injury that should heal with time. As the tenderness diminishes, you will need to stretch the muscles in front of your leg. This can best be done by lunges.

While recuperating from this injury, and as you begin activity, stretch and heat this area before activity. If it hurts, you probably still need more time to heal.

Football players often incur this injury many times during a game. To return players to the game, physicians inject corticosteroid. This can alleviate the pain, but it can actually cause deterioration of the tendon.

Hip pointers are different from avulsion fractures of the anterior superior iliac spine. However, they can occur in the same way and produce pain in the same area. Fractures are bone breaks resulting from the tendon of the sartorius muscle pulling the bone off at its insertion.

Hip pointers occur more often in adolescents than in adults. An x-ray can help a physician make the diagnosis.

QUADRICEP PULLS

The muscles in front of your leg can also sustain a strain or partial tear, usually at the musculoskeletal junction. You will experience pain but will not have swelling. With severe strains, your leg may turn black and blue. Applying ice will help initially. After the first twenty-four hours, your thigh will feel stiff.

Begin heating and mild stretching exercises only after forty-eight hours.

Hamstring Pulls

The muscles in the back of your leg can also sustain a strain. The area that becomes injured may be in the middle of the back of your leg.

More often, however, the injury occurs where the muscle inserts into the bone of your pelvis. This area is the bone on which you sit.

If this is an acute injury, resting and applying ice will help. The gradual institution of stretching exercises should also help. The best way to stretch these muscles is to touch your toes with your legs straight while in both sitting and standing positions. Heating before activity is also an option.

Like the muscles in the front of your leg, the tendon of the hamstring muscles can occasionally pull off a piece of bone. This injury occurs more often with adolescents. An x-ray can help a physician make a diagnosis.

This is a common injury among runners, sprinters, and football players. Thoroughly stretching before activity can help to prevent this injury.

Groin (Adductor) Pulls

Groin pulls are strains of the adductor muscles that insert into the pubis bone. These muscles include the adductor magnus, longus, and brevis. Your adductor longus is most often the muscle that you pull.

This injury occurs when one leg travels too far away from the other, away from the midline, like when you do a split. Football players, gymnasts, and soccer players are most at risk for this injury due to the nature of their sports.

Groin pulls can be quite severe, sometimes with much bruising in the groin area. This black and blue can sometimes travel down the length of your leg.

If you sustain this injury, rest and apply ice initially. Gradual stretching exercises will help you return to sports.

You may require crutches because the pain can be quite disabling. With proper rest and stretching, you should heal in about two to six weeks.

For Strains, DO

❖ Rest.

❖ Apply ice the first twenty-four to forty-eight hours.

❖ Stretch and apply heat only after the first forty-eight hours.

For Strains, DO NOT

❖ Apply heat in the first twenty-four to forty eight hours.

❖ Stretch in the first twenty-four hours.

❖ Use an anti-inflammatory medication.

For Strains, Red Flags

❖ Severe black and blue.

❖ Not healing within the first week.

❖ All muscle strains should heal, if treated properly, within six weeks.

THE HIP

Bursitis

When you participate in any type of activity that repetitively uses the muscles around your hip, you can sustain an inflammation of one of the two major bursae of your hip. These bursae are the greater trochanteric and the ischial bursa.

The greater trochanteric bursa is located on a ridge of bone found mid-way between your front and back pants pockets. The ischial bursa is at the ridge of bone that comes into contact with a chair when you sit.

If you have inflammation of either of these bursae, known as bursitis, you will feel pain with hip movement. In addition, you may feel pain when you sit on a chair.

Resting and applying ice will help. In addition, you can immediately use an anti-inflammatory medication if you can tolerate aspirin.

DO

❖ Rest.

❖ Apply ice.

❖ Use an anti-inflammatory medication.

❖ Use crutches.

DO NOT

❖ Continue participation.

❖ Use heat.

RED FLAGS

❖ Not healing within the first week.

SNAPPING HIP CONDITIONS

SARTORIUS IMPINGEMENT SYNDROME

A rare condition called sartorius impingement syndrome can cause hip pain. The sartorius is a muscle that attaches just in front of your hip and toward your groin in the area near your front pants pocket.

When you place your hand into your pocket, leaving your thumb on the outside, your thumb points to a ridge of bone on your pelvis. This is not actually your hip bone but your pelvis bone. The ridge of bone is called the anterior superior iliac spine, one attachment of the sartorius muscle. This muscle travels down your leg and inserts on the inside of your knee on the lower leg bone or tibia.

Near the sartorius tendon, the cable that attaches the muscle to the bone is a bursa or sac that allows the tendon to move in close proximity to your pelvis. This tendon can occasionally slip over the bursa and surround the bone, resulting in a pop and sometimes pain.

This injury usually occurs during internal and external rotation of the hip with the hip fully flexed. Some of my patients have told me that this injury usually occurs when they try to stand after sitting Indian style, a position with the hip fully flexed and completely externally rotated.

If your hips are wide and you have knock-knees, or if you have congenital dislocation of the hip (CDH), you may be more predisposed to this injury than other people. Gymnasts can experience this injury since they are often in extreme positions.

OTHER CONDITIONS

Other structures around your hip that can snap with movement include your iliotibial band, iliofemoral ligaments, and biceps femoris tendon. You do not need to differentiate which of these structures is causing your injury in order to begin some self-care.

DO

❖   Rest.

❖   Apply ice.

❖   Use an anti-inflammatory medication if you can take aspirin.

DO NOT

❖   Continue to perform movements that cause pain.

❖   Apply heat.

With time, this injury will usually heal on its own. The injury does not occur frequently or repetitively. Avoid moving into positions that cause the injury. If you continue to have pain consult a physician. In the meantime, continue stretching and try to rest. Anti-inflammatory medication can also help.

RED FLAGS

❖   No relief from pain within one week.

❖   Continued snapping.

MISCELLANEOUS HIP CONDITIONS

The following conditions can either be congenital, resulting from birth defects, or acquired. Most of these can cause severe injuries to your hips if they are untreated. Avoid impact type activity if you have such injuries.

CONGENITAL DISLOCATION OF THE HIP (CDH)

CDH, now called developmental dysplasia of the hip (DDH), is a developmental problem affecting the hips at birth. Females are more predisposed to this problem than males. Doctors routinely examine newborns for this condition. On occasion, however, especially in medically underserved areas of the country, doctors fail to diagnose the injury.

The condition ranges from slight dislocation or subluxation to actual dislocation of the hip. This occurs because the roof of the hip joint or the hip bone itself does not develop normally. If you are born with this problem and are not treated, you may develop early arthritis of your hip.

If you live with this condition, avoid such repetitive, heavy impact activities as aerobics and basketball.

AVASCULAR NECROSIS

Avascular necrosis of the hip (AVN) is an acquired condition. Alcohol consumption, blood dyscrasias (imbalance of the constituents of the blood or bone marrow), deep diving, and sickle cell anemia can cause (AVN). Your hip bone does not receive enough blood, so parts of your hip bone die.

SLIPPED CAPITAL FEMORAL EPIPHYSIS

Slipped capital femoral epiphysis is a congenital condition that can cause your hip bones to separate or fracture. Consult an orthopaedist regarding this condition.

LEGG-CALVE-PERTHES DISEASE

Legg-Calve-perthes disease is a congenital condition

similar to acquired AVN. The same principles of AVN treatment apply. In addition, a child or adolescent with this condition should be treated by an orthopaedist.

CHAPTER 18:

THE BACK AND NECK

THE BACK

The spinal column is similar in construction in both the neck and lower back. The two areas are vastly different, however, in their function. The neck is more responsible for allowing a wide range of motion while the lower back experiences great force through it.

Vertebrae are blocks of bone lined up on top of each other. Between the vertebrae are discs that serve as shock absorbers. Motion can occur through the disc segments.

Motion also can occur through small facet joints that are anatomically similar to a knee joint. They have a capsule with a small amount of fluid. They move forward and backward and side to side and have a rotational capability.

Surrounding the spine, or the blocks of vertebrae, are ligaments that hold the vertebrae together. Muscles also help move the spine and support it. The muscles of both the back and the chest also support and stabilize the spine.

Your abdominal muscles support the spine by increasing hydrostatic pressure. They compress your abdomen that then acts like a waterbed to compress the vertebrae.

Spine injuries can affect any of the above structures. Any sports activity that places increased pressure on the vertebrae and discs can, in conjunction with a rotatory force, injure the above structures. Sprains of the ligaments, strains of the muscles, herniations of the discs, tears in the covering of the disc, and injuries to the facet joints can occur.

Regardless of the type of injury, you may experience back pain. The back muscles may go into spasms. You may occasionally have pain in your buttocks and the posterior part of your hip. The pain can also be in your leg, primarily in the back part of the thigh.

In rare cases, the pain may shoot down your leg to the toes. If this occurs, this is a serious problem because you have probably injured your shock absorber.

In addition to pain, you may experience numbness, tingling, and the strange sensation of warm or cold water running down your leg. The muscles in your leg may also twitch continually.

STRAINS

Strains can be quite debilitating. You can strain your back in any sport. The strain may be so severe that you are unable to move. Strains, however, generally heal with a short period of rest.

DISC AND NERVE INJURIES

More severe back injuries are those that disrupt the shock absorbing function of the discs. The nerves that exit your spinal column run quite close to the discs. Injuries to discs can be a simple tear of the outer covering or a tear that allows the gelatinous shock absorber to seep out.

Both injuries can cause back and leg pain, as well as numbness and tingling in the leg. If you have weakness of a muscle in your lower extremity, you have probably herniated the disc. The fragment that has seeped out is pressing on a nerve.

You may, instead, experience tingling and pain that move down the back side of the leg but not past the knee. In this case, you have probably torn the covering of the disc but not allowed a fragment to seep out.

Some anatomic factors can cause these injuries. Tight hamstring muscles can predispose you to back injury, as can an arched lower back.

PREVENTION

❖ Stretch your hamstrings.
❖ Stretch your back.
❖ Strengthen your back muscles.
❖ Strengthen your abdomen.

TECHNIQUE MODIFICATIONS

❖ Avoid too much forward or backward motion.
❖ Know and use proper technique.

RED FLAGS

❖ Back pain
❖ Leg pain
❖ Toe numbness
❖ Inability to lift your big toe
❖ Inability to lift your ankle
❖ A continuous muscle twitch

<u>THE NECK</u>

While the neck is not subjected to too much body weight, great force can still be transmitted through this area. The neck can sustain injuries like those experienced in the lower spine.

Football players can sustain injuries called stingers that often occur during tackles. The injury causes pain, tingling, or numbness in one or both arms. See the information about stingers in the chapter on football in Part I.

Coaches teach players to hit with their head upright. This is important because when you hit someone with the crown of your head, your neck feels a great force.

The neck normally has some lordosis, which is the type of curvature found in the neck of a swan. If you hit with your head straight, that is with the crown of your head, the vertebrae can all pile up on each other. When you make contact, the neck is forced forward and this can disrupt the discs. This motion may place too much pressure on the nerves and cause pain, numbness, or tingling.

This injury can cause you to stop play for a day or, in extreme cases, it can end one's football career. Players who repeatedly sustain this injury are at risk for severe spinal cord injury. Consider professional consultation regarding all neck injuries.

CHAPTER 19:

THE SHOULDER AND ARM

The shoulder and arm are often injured in sporting activities that require the arm to be brought above the head. Such activities include baseball, racquetball, squash, swimming, tennis, and volleyball.

THE SHOULDER

The shoulder, unlike the knee, allows a great range of motion. The shoulder socket, however, is quite shallow. Most of the shoulder's stability comes from the surrounding soft tissue structures. The shoulder has to be able to place itself in extreme positions and with precise placement, particularly in athletes who move their arms over their head.

The shoulder is an interesting joint. Not only does it have a shallow socket but the ball (humeral head) and socket have a roof of bone over them, the acromion. Thus, when the arm moves, it must move completely below a ledge of bone. Between the ledge and the ball portion of your shoulder lie the bursae and the rotator cuff.

TYPES OF INJURIES

You may wonder why the ball portion of your shoulder does not run into the roof bone when you raise your hand over your head. This occurs because of your rotator cuff, a combination of four tendons between the ball of the shoulder joint and the roof bone. The rotator cuff not only helps your arm move, it keeps the ball portion of your shoulder in place and down and away from the roof of the bone.

IMPINGEMENT

Shoulder impingement pain occurs when the ball in the socket of the shoulder joint runs into the roof of bone. There are many causes of this injury, but I will describe the effects of the injury.

Between the ball in the socket of the shoulder joint and the roof of bone lie the rotator cuff and the shoulder bursae. When you compress the ball into the roof, squeezing the rotator cuff and bursae, you cause damage to these structures.

The tissues then become inflamed, which is the body's way of trying to heal the damaged area. The inflammation is quite painful.

The bursae, containing a sac of fluid, can also become inflamed. They then fill with water. You may experience a sensation of something being crunched in your shoulder. Patients often comment that they have "rice-crispies" in their shoulder.

Thus, with impingement, the rotator cuff can neither help your arm move nor hold the ball portion of the socket down and away from the roof bone. It loses its ability to control the ball in the socket when it becomes inflamed or torn. Chronic inflammation of the rotator cuff can cause it to wear.

Always consult an orthopaedist regarding shoulder pain. If you have an inflamed shoulder, you might first try to decrease the inflammation. Then try to strengthen the front and back muscles of the rotator cuff. This may sound simple, but it is difficult to avoid recurring inflammation.

Rest, use an anti-inflammatory medication, and perform some stretching exercises. When your shoulder becomes inflamed, the back portion of your shoulder typically feels tight. When this occurs, your injury thrusts the shoulder forward and causes the ball to run into the roof of bone.

To prevent this injury, stretch out the back portion of your shoulder. Place the affected extremity on the wall. For example, if your right shoulder hurts, place your shoulder, elbow and wrist on the wall. Without allowing either of them to leave the wall, face the wall with both feet facing forward.

Lean forward to try to touch your unaffected shoulder to the elbow of the affected side now on the wall. This exercise is done at the level of your stomach, breast, and eyes.

Shoulder pain is quite debilitating for athletes who throw overhead. You should seek treatment by an orthopaedic surgeon well trained in shoulder injuries.

To prevent shoulder impingement, always stretch and warm up prior to any throwing activity. Especially stretch the back portion of your shoulder joint. You should also make sure the muscles in the front and back of your shoulder are strong since they help to hold the ball in your shoulder joint's socket down and away from the roof of bone.

Biceps Tendonitis

Another common shoulder injury among throwing athletes is that to the tendons of the biceps that are located in the shoulder and the elbow.

The biceps tendon is connected to the shoulder joint and inserts into the upper portion of the glenoid rim inside your shoulder. If you have inflammation of this tendon, you will have pain in the front portion of your shoulder. You can prevent this injury by stretching your biceps prior to throwing.

Prevention

  ❖ Stretch your shoulder, especially the posterior capsule.
  ❖ Strengthen the front and back muscles of your rotator cuff.
  ❖ Use proper form when playing.
  ❖ Rest when you are fatigued.

TECHNIQUE MODIFICATION

* Avoid throwing sidearm.
* While doing the crawl stroke in swimming, make sure your arm exits the water completely and is placed properly into the water on re-enrty.
* When spiking a ball in volleyball, make sure your shoulder is directly behind the ball.
* When playing tennis or racquetball, serve or smash from directly behind the ball, not from the side.

RED FLAGS

* Any shoulder pain that persists after a week of rest.

THE ARM

Few athletic injuries directly affect the arm. Most of the pain comes from injuries to the shoulder, elbow, or biceps tendon. About the only arm injury that does occur, especially with baseball players, is a stress fracture of the arm.

Upper arm pain usually comes from your shoulder. Lower arm pain usually comes from your elbow or biceps tendon.

CHAPTER 20:

THE FOREARM AND ELBOW

Most forearm and elbow pain from athletic injury comes from the inflammation of tendons. The pain usually occurs because you are overdoing the activity. Athletes, especially pitchers, can disrupt the ligaments that hold the upper arm to the lower arm. The nerves in the arm can also become inflamed.

LIGAMENT DISRUPTIONS

In addition to the flexor-pronator muscle masses, the elbow has the medial collateral ligament that holds the upper arm bone to the lower arm bone. This ligament can rupture.

With repetitive throwing, athletes can tear this ligament. Baseball pitchers are especially susceptible to this injury.

Pitchers should use the techniques I suggested earlier for tendonitis injuries. If the injury remains, consult an orthopaedic surgeon.

A cortisone injection is sometimes needed. Have it administered by an orthopaedic surgeon familiar with the anatomy in this area. Avoid having more than one shot.

PREVENTION

❖ Stretch well.
❖ Strengthen your muscles.
❖ Use anti-inflammatories.

❖ Warm up well.
TECHNIQUE MODIFICATION
❖ Throw overhand, not sidearm.
❖ Use a mild stretching program.

RED FLAGS
❖ Any pain that persists after a week of rest

NERVE IRRITATIONS

ULNAR NERVE, CUBITAL TUNNEL SYNDROME

The ulnar nerve in the middle of your elbow can become irritated. If you have ever hit your funny bone, you have found your ulnar nerve.

Inflammation of this nerve can occur if you engage in too much typing, or sleeping with your elbow flexed. Ulnar nerve injury occurs quite frequently among pitchers.

If you have been unsuccessful in reducing the inflammation, stretch your elbow and sleep with your arms straight. The nerve can become so irritated that it needs to be moved around in front of the elbow.

RADIAL NERVE

Another is the radial nerve on the back side of the forearm. This nerve can become compressed when the muscles work overtime.

The pain from this injury feels like that of a tennis elbow. Consult an orthopaedic surgeon for an accurate diagnosis.

TENDONITIS

Tendons in your arm connect muscles to bones. There are three places at which tendons inserted into your arm can become inflamed and cause pain. Remember, however, that pain on the outside of your arm and about half-way up usually comes from your shoulder.

TENNIS ELBOW

One area where tendons are inserted into the arm is on the outside of your arm near the elbow. The muscles are called the extensor mass. Tennis elbow injuries occur when you have one specific place where there is extreme tenderness. If you are a right-handed tennis player, you usually feel the pain when the ball makes contact with your racquet on a backhand swing. This pain can be debilitating and cause you to cease your sport.

You need to prevent this injury. During the preseason, strengthen your elbow muscles by stretching.

Tennis elbow can also be sustained by computer users, typists, and golfers. If you sustain it, cease your activity. Next try to decrease the inflammation at the tendon site with anti-inflammatory medications. However, be aware that such medications can upset your stomach.

Once the pain begins to subside, you can perform some simple stretching. Then try to do some strengthening. If you can do so without pain, you can then try your activity again.

You can also try to use a tennis elbow strap. Tie it tightly around your forearm. The strap causes the force usually felt by the tendons to be absorbed through the strap, not transmitted to the bony insertion site.

GOLFER'S ELBOW

A second area where there are tendons that can become inflamed in a similar way is on the inside of your elbow. This group of muscles is called the flexor-pronator mass medial epicondylitis.

This injury is sometimes known as golfer's elbow. This injury is an inflammation of these muscles and tendons. Prevention and treatment are similar to those for tendonitis.

OTHER INJURIES

The area directly in front of your elbow crease to slightly below it is a third place where a tendon can become inflamed. Baseball pitchers commonly experience this injury. This is where your biceps tendon inserts.

Prevention of this injury begins with an effective stretching and strengthening program. If you have pain and have tried all the methods described above to reduce it, try sleeping with your arm as straight as possible. You will have a tendency when you sleep to lie in the fetal position. This, however, allows the biceps tendon to shorten. You may need to sleep with a splint to keep your arm completely extended. If you do this and still have pain, consult an orthopaedist.

CHAPTER 21:

THE HAND AND WRIST

The hand can be injured with almost any sport. Athletes whose sport involves the use of a ball are most susceptible to this injury.

Hand injuries occur when athletes who are concentrating on the ball become tired or distracted and do not properly receive the ball.

TYPES OF INJURIES

FRACTURES AND DISLOCATIONS

When you catch a ball incorrectly, you can sustain a jammed finger, one of the most common injuries. Most jammed finger injuries do not result in tears of the surrounding hand ligaments holding together the small bones of the wrist and fingers. However, such ligaments can be stressed.

If the ball hits the tips of the fingers or the thumb, it can place pressure on the joint, which causes pain. You can experience severe pain that can prevent you from playing your sport.

If you have not already broken a bone or torn a ligament, a simple and quick remedy is to apply ice until the fingers become numb. You can buddy tape one finger to the other. The tape may, however, interfere with your ability to play the sport.

If your finger jam injury is severe, you may sustain a fracture of the bones in your finger. You can also dislocate a bone. Both of these injuries are serious.

Your coach or athletic trainer on the field may reduce the pain of a fracture. However, have an orthopaedic surgeon examine these injuries. There is often much more damage than is apparent.

Hand dislocations and fractures can be treated by splinting and surgical means. Such injuries should be treated professionally since you want to have motion when your injuries have healed.

TENDON RUPTURES AND INFLAMMATION

Several tendons extend from the muscles in your forearm to the bones in your wrist, hand, and fingers. With continued use, any of these tendons can become inflamed.

Tendons are like cables enclosed within sheaths that connect muscles to bones. Think of tendons as the line on a fishing pole and the sheaths as the eyelets through which the fishing line is strung. The sheaths, however, are quite a bit thicker and wider than the eyelets on a fishing pole.

Tendons lie near bones and can become irritated on the bone. When tears occur, the tendons become inflamed and cause pain. Some swelling can also occur because of fluid accumulating in the area.

The primary treatment is to rest the involved body part and take anti-inflammatory medications. You can then begin stretching out these tendons. They can become scarred next to the sheath during inflammation.

After stretching thoroughly, slowly try to increase the strength of the muscles attached to the affected tendons. This can help prevent reinjury.

Tendons can rupture as a result of great force. You will have pain and an immediate loss of movement. Fingers are also likely to be affected and will not function properly. Consult an orthopaedic surgeon immediately.

LIGAMENT DISRUPTIONS

You can rupture your tendons when you receive a direct blow from an object. Such injuries can be quite debilitating. Some disruptions may not heal unless they are properly splinted.

One common example of a ligament disruption is skier's thumb. Those who snow ski with their wrist through the strap on the ski pole and then fall and catch their pole in the snow are susceptible to this injury. They rupture the ligament that holds the thumb bone together.

The thumb ligament is known not to heal too well. When the thumb ligament tears, it moves from its normal position, and another structure falls in the way to prevent its healing.

If you sustain any ligament injury, that can occur with any dislocation or a jammed finger injury, consult an orthopaedic surgeon.

NERVE COMPRESSIONS

Any of the three nerves that extend across the wrist can become compressed by the overlying ligament and inflamed. Carpal tunnel syndrome, for instance, results from inflammation of the median nerve, the major nerve on the palm side of the hand.

Numbness or tingling in the thumb, the index finger, and the middle finger can result from compression. If this injury is left untreated, it can produce pain and weakness in your hand and eventually muscle wasting.

Resting, using splints, and taking anti-inflammatory medications can help reduce the symptoms if you begin them early enough. With chronic problems, surgery is sometimes recommended. The median nerve extends in a tunnel that can become compressed by the overlying ligament. Surgery consists of releasing the ligament.

Also avoid sleeping in the fetal position with your wrists bent. This simply compresses the nerves, which aggravates the injury.

GANGLIONS

Ganglions are small hard balls of tissue that appear around your wrist. They can be quite painful. Around your wrists and hands are a number of small bones connected by ligaments and encased by capsules. The capsules have valves that lead into small sacs. When the sacs become inflamed and fluid is produced, they can fill and produce pain. This is how ganglions develop.

Ganglions may appear and disappear. In earlier times, physicians advised patients to hit the sacs with a book to rupture them. That was sometimes effective, but the ganglions generally returned. If you have painful ganglions that do not diminish with rest, you can have them removed.

PREVENTION

❖ Stretch well before activity.

TECHNIQUE MODIFICATION

❖ Concentrate on catching the ball.
❖ Be aware when you are tired.
❖ Strengthen the muscles you use for your sport.
❖ Consider taping your fingers before you play, if you are prone to jamming them.

RED FLAGS

❖ Any finger, hand, or wrist injury that does not heal within one week.

APPENDIX A

SPORTS MEDICINE SOCIETIES

MAJOR SOCIETIES

There are three major national-level sports medicine societies in the United States. They are the American College of Sports Medicine (ACSM), the American Medical Society for Sports Medicine (AMSSM), and the American Orthopaedic Society for Sports Medicine (AOSSM).

The ACSM, an affiliate of the Federation Internationale de Medicine Sportive, serves members who include athletic team physicians, orthopaedic surgeons, athletic trainers, and others concerned with the effects of sports and exercise on health.

The AMSSM, an affiliate of the American Osteopathic Association, provides education for its member physicians who include primary care, non-surgical sports medicine physicians.

The AOSSM, whose members must be orthopaedists, promotes the prevention, recognition, and orthopaedic treatment of sports injuries. It educates members by providing postgraduate courses in a cooperative effort with the American Academy of Orthopaedic Surgeons (AAOS). In cooperation with the AMSSM, it educates athletic team physicians by offering such courses as Current Concepts and Controversies for the Team Physician. The organization works closely with the Team Physician Society of the National Football League.

These three organizations differ in their focus and membership but all work together. They work closely with the Orthopaedic Research and Education Foundation (OREF) and the Foundation for Sportsmedicine and Education (FSME). Which are affiliated with the American Academy of Orthopaedic Surgeons (AAOS).

OTHER SOCIETIES

Non-physicians who are involved in sports medicine can join other societies, as well. These include the National Athletic Trainers Association (NATA) and the Sports Physical Therapy Association (SPTA).

Non-orthopaedists can obtain added training in sports medicine by performing clerkships offered by various independent sponsors.

American College of Sports Medicine (ACSM) National Center
Box 1440, Indianapolis, IN 46206-1440
(317) 637-9200 ~ (317) 634-7817 Fax
Founded in 1954

American Medical Society for Sports Medicine (AMSSM)
7611 Elmwood Avenue, Suite 201, Middletown, WI 52562-0623
(608) 831-4484 ~ (608) 831-5122
Founded in 1975

American Orthopaedic Society for Sports Medicine (AOSSM)
6300 N. River Road, Suite 200, Rosemont, IL 60018-4229
(708) 292-4900 ~ (708) 292-4905 fax
Founded in 1972

American Academy of Orthopaedic Surgeons
6300 N. River Road, Rosemont, IL 60018-4262
(708) 823-7186 ~ (708) 823-8125 Fax
Founded in 1933

The National Athletic Trainers' Association (NATA)
2952 Stemmons Parkway, Suite 200, Dallas, TX 75247
(214) 637-6282 ~ (214) 637-2206 Fax
Founded in 1950

The Sports Physical Therapy Section of The American Physical Therapy Association (SPTA)
1111 N. Fairfax Street, Alexandria, VA 22314-1488
(703) 684-2782 ~ (703) 684-7343 Fax
Founded in 1921

APPEDIX B

EDUCATION REQUIREMENTS FOR DIFFERENT TYPES OF DOCTORS

Minimum Undergraduate Requirements, In Years, For Different Types Of Doctors

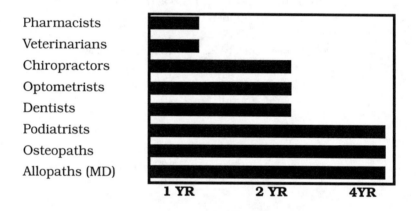

Professional School Training For Different Types Of Doctors

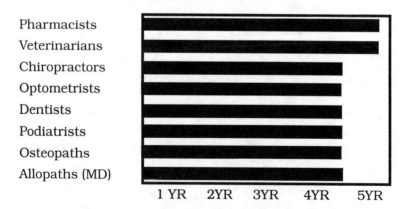

* DISCLAIMER - The values used in this graph were obtained from career pamphlet information sources and are used to generalize for the purpose of graphic illustration.

Potential Years Of Internship/Residency For Doctors

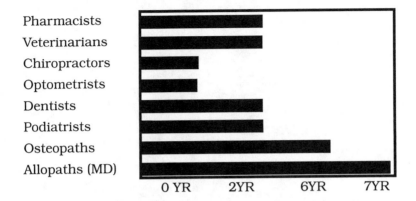

Years After Professional School For Licensing And Certification

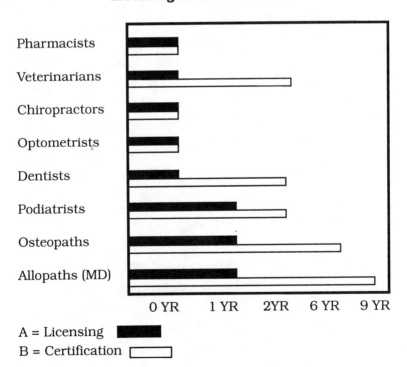

A = Licensing
B = Certification

* DISCLAIMER - The values used in this graph were obtained from career pamphlet information sources and are used to generalize for the purpose of graphic illustration.

Index

ABOUT THE AUTHOR

William F. Bennett, M.D. is an orthopaedic surgeon specializing in orthopaedic sports medicine. He has also participated in athletics all his life as both a national competitor and recreational athlete.

Dr. Bennett maintains a private practice in orthopaedic surgery, with subspecialization training in sportsmedicine and in shoulder surgery, in Sarasota, Florida. He provides both surgical and non-surgical treatment to patients of all ages and athletic abilities, with injuries to any body part.

He is also the founder and Chief Executive Officer of the Florida Orthopaedic and Sports Medicine Institute (FOSMI).

Dr. Bennett has developed new surgical techniques in ankle surgery. In addition, he has published articles in scholarly journals for physicians, as well as for orthopaedic surgeons. He remains active in research and teaching.

He is licensed to practice medicine in Florida, California, and Texas.

Dr. Bennett completed his subspecialization training in Switzerland with Christian Gerber, M.D., world renowned shoulder expert, and in California where he completed an orthopaedic sports medicine fellowship at the Los Angeles Orthopaedic Institute. He completed an orthopaedic surgery residency at the University of South Florida Medical School in Tampa and at the University of Texas Health Science Center at the Texas Medical Center in Houston.

Prior to that time, he completed a general surgery internship at the Baylor University Medical Center in Dallas, Texas. His medical school education was completed at the University of Connecticut Health Science Center in Farmington, Connecticut.

Dr. Bennett graduated Phi Beta Kappa and Magna Cum Laude, with honors, from Wake Forest University in Winston Salem, North Carolina with a B.S. degree.

Dr. Bennett is a long-time wrestler, having been a Connecticut State Wrestling Champion and an Amateur Athletic Union National Junior Olympic Championship Qualifier. He is also a proficient water-skier.

BACKGROUND
WILLIAM F. BENNETT, M.D.
ORTHOPAEDIC SURGEON

SUBSPECIALTIES:
SPORTSMEDICINE/ARTHROSCOPY/LASER SURGERY
SHOULDER/KNEE/HIP/ELBOW SURGERY

Dr. William F. Bennett specializes in the diagnosis and treatment of all musculoskeletal disorders, including afflictions of the shoulder, knee, hip, elbow, hand, wrist, ankle, foot and spine in children and adults. He routinely performs total joint replacements of the shoulder, knee and hip. He is an expert in arthroscopic treatment of conditions involving the shoulder, knee and ankle.

Dr. Bennett has received extensive training in minimally invasive surgery, arthroscopic and laser surgery which has enabled him to treat highly competitive athletes, and return them to their previous levels of competition. Dr. Bennett, however, does not limit his practice to competitive athletes, and treats all patients with the aim of returning them to functional activity with efficient medical and limited surgical intervention. His surgical skills are swift, efficient and technically precise. With total knee replacements his patients are usually off the operating table in 45-60 minutes, lessening the risks of any and all complications. He is published extensively on disorders of the musculoskeletal system in leading medical journals. He lectures nationally on musculoskeletal disease, particularly the shoulder and the knee, and is the founder of **FOSMI, The Florida Orthopaedic and Sportsmedicine Institute** in Sarasota, Florida, his chosen home.

Dr. Bennett is Board Certified by the American Board of Orthopaedic Surgeons (ABOS), is a member of the American Academy of Orthopaedic Surgeons (AAOS), and the Arthroscopy Association of North America (AANA).

FOSMI
The Florida Orthopaedic and Sportsmedicine Institute

Dr. William F. Bennett founded the Florida Orthopedic and Sportsmedicine Institute (FOSMI) in 1995. At FOSMI we have a group of highly trained subspecialists who treat musculoskeletal injuries with up-to-date, state-of-the-art technology. FOSMI provides this service not only to the inhabitants of the west coast of Florida, but also to patients who travel long distances across the United States and from abroad for treatment. We have had patients from as far away as Phoenix, Arizona, and Hungary have visited our institute. The physicians here at FOSMI can speak French and Italian. The physicians at FOSMI have trained at some of the best training programs in the world. This affords patients immediate and definitive diagnoses. Most of the conditions seen here are initially treated nonsurgically. However, as a tertiary referral center, we often are referred patients who need surgery. If surgery is required for your condition, our surgeons are trained with minimally invasive techniques like arthroscopy and laser surgery to set you on the road to recovery quicker and more efficiently than conventional open techniques.

FOSMI is an organization which has its focus in patient care and education. The educational focus lies not only in educating other orthopaedic surgeons and physicians about advances in the treatment of musculoskeletal disease, by writing scientific papers and presenting lectures at national forums, but by educating you, the patient, about your condition. The physicians and surgeons at FOSMI do this by creating an open-door policy. Before you leave the office you should be satisfied that a proper working diagnosis has been formulated for your problem and any questions regarding your condition have been answered to your satisfaction.

You will notice when you visit FOSMI, the office is constructed in an open and friendly manner, to alleviate any anxiety you may have.

STATE OF THE ART TECHNOLOGY

If surgery is needed for your condition, Dr. Bennett has the ability to treat most conditions of your shoulder, knee or ankle with an Arthroscope. An arthroscope is a small telescope with which surgeons can view the inside of your knee, elbow, shoulder, ankle or wrist joint. By using this fiber optic device and viewing your joint problem on a monitor (like a television screen), our surgeons, with the aid of other small arthroscopic and laser tools can treat your problem.

Not all conditions can be treated with an arthroscope-- severe disabling arthritis of the knee, shoulder and hip are conditions which are not amenable to arthroscopic interv- ention. Should you need a joint replacement, our surgeons here are FOSMI are also adept and technically proficient with these procedures.

One of the most recent advances in arthroscopic surgery, and a technique which is employed at only a few institutions in the United States, is an arthroscopic rotator cuff repair. This approach also allows you to return to a functional status in about one third of the time it would take if your shoulder were to be opened.

Please contact our office for futher information:
Florida Orthopaedic and Sportsmedicine Institute (FOSMI)
Sarasota Medical Center
5741 Bee Ridge Road, Suite 470
Sarasota, Florida 34233 USA
(941) 379-5509 ~ (941) 379-5713 fax
E-mail: orthsurg@aol.com or Compuserve 104421.3453
Internet: www.investors.org/fosmi

"THE ATHLETE IN YOU" MAKES A GREAT GIFT FOR ANYONE WHO PARTICIPATES IN SPORTS.

☎ Call us toll free at: (800) 307-0001
   Fax us at: (941) 953-3915

✉ Mail order to: Pinnacle Press at
   P.O. Box 2787, Sarasota, FL 34230-2787

🖥 On-line orders: E-Mail Pinnacle Press at:
   pci@smallbizz.org or on the Internet at
   www.smallbizz.org/pci/

Quantity	Name of Book*	Price

* The Athlete In You $ 12.95
* The Joy of Self-Employment, Todd L. Mayo $ 27.95
* Pathways to Success, Todd L. Mayo $14.95

Florida residents please add 7% sales tax to your order.	**Subtotal** _____
	Sales tax _____
Surface Shipping & Handling is $3.95 for first book and $1.00 for each add'l book. Air shipping is $5.00 for each book.	**S & H** _____
	Total _____

Name: _____

Address: _____

City:_____**State:**_____ **Zip:**_____

Telephone: _____

Credit Card: _____

Account #: _____

Name as it appears on the card: _____

Signature:_____

☐   **Check Enclosed**

"THE ATHLETE IN YOU" MAKES A GREAT GIFT FOR ANYONE WHO PARTICIPATES IN SPORTS.

Call us toll free at: (800) 307-0001
Fax us at: (941) 953-3915

Mail order to: Pinnacle Press at
P.O. Box 2787, Sarasota, FL 34230-2787

On-line orders: E-Mail Pinnacle Press at:
pci@smallbizz.org or on the Internet at
www.smallbizz.org/pci/

Quantity	Name of Book*	Price

* The Athlete In You $ 12.95
* The Joy of Self-Employment, Todd L. Mayo $ 27.95
* Pathways to Success, Todd L. Mayo $14.95

Florida residents please add 7% sales tax to your order. Surface Shipping & Handling is $3.95 for first book and $1.00 for each add'l book. Air shipping is $5.00 for each book.	**Subtotal** _____ **Sales tax** _____ **S & H** _____ **Total** _____

Name: _____

Address: _____

City: _____ **State:** _____ **Zip:** _____

Telephone: _____

Credit Card: _____

Account #: _____

Name as it appears on the card: _____

Signature: _____

☐   **Check Enclosed**